Creating Conditions

Based on original ethnographic research, this monograph examines the impact of new genetic knowledge on the classification of one syndrome to illuminate more general issues concerning the construction and interpretation of diseases and syndromes. It follows the work of clinicians, scientists, activists, parents and others to understand the trajectory of a genetic condition. This is an especially timely exercise. As one among a vast number of conditions that have been associated with genetic causes, Rett syndrome illustrates some of the most significant developments in contemporary medicine. While the impacts of genetics on contemporary medicine are many and diverse, the identification of conditions as genetic is a significant feature of current medical thought and perception. This monograph provides a key exemplar of the implications of genetic medicine that are far-reaching and extend well beyond this particular syndrome.

This multi-sited ethnography follows the phenomenon across various key encounters and institutional contexts to illustrate the multiple circuits and sites where relationships between research, diagnosis, treatment and social mobilization take place. These are by no means linear processes. The laboratory and the clinic, the family and the support-group are all subject to mutual influence and this monograph documents the multiple sites and versions in which this medical condition is enacted and represented.

Katie Featherstone is Senior Lecturer within the Cardiff School of Nursing and Midwifery and a Research Fellow at Cesagen, Cardiff University. A sociologist of medicine, her recent ethnographic work includes an examination of the social consequences and clinical utilization of new genetic technologies, specifically within dysmorphology, a specialism of clinical genetics, and an examination of kinship and disclosure in the context of genetic information (The Wellcome Trust).

Paul Atkinson is Distinguished Research Professor of Sociology at Cardiff University. He is an Academician of the Academy of Social Sciences. Recent publications include *Everyday Arias: An Operatic Ethnography* and *Contours of Culture*, with Sara Delamont and William Housley. Together with Sara Delamont he edits the journal *Qualitative Research*. He is currently conducting ethnographic work in art-makers' studios.

Genetics and Society

Series Editors: Ruth Chadwick, *Director of Cesagen, Cardiff University*; John Dupré, *Director of Egenis, Exeter University*; David Wield, *Director of Innogen, Edinburgh University*; and Steve Yearley, *Director of the Genomics Forum, Edinburgh University.*

The books in this series, all based on original research, explore the social, economic and ethical consequences of the new genetic sciences. The series is based in the Cesagen, one of the centres forming the ESRC's Genomics Network (EGN), the largest UK investment in social-science research on the implications of these innovations. With a mix of research monographs, edited collections, textbooks and a major new handbook, the series is a valuable contribution to the social analysis of developing and emergent biotechnologies.
Series titles include:

New Genetics, New Social Formations
Peter Glasner, Paul Atkinson and Helen Greenslade

New Genetics, New Identities
Paul Atkinson, Peter Glasner and Helen Greenslade

The GM Debate
Risk, politics and public engagement
Tom Horlick-Jones, John Walls, Gene Rowe, Nick Pidgeon, Wouter Poortinga, Graham Murdock and Tim O'Riordan

Growth Cultures
Life sciences and economic development
Philip Cooke

Human Cloning in the Media
Joan Haran, Jenny Kitzinger, Maureen McNeil and Kate O'Riordan

Local Cells, Global Science
Embryonic stem cell research in India
Aditya Bharadwaj and Peter Glasner

Handbook of Genetics and Society
Paul Atkinson, Peter Glasner and Margaret Lock

The Human Genome
Chamundeeswari Kuppuswamy

Community Genetics and Genetic Alliances
Eugenics, carrier testing and networks of risk
Aviad E. Raz

Neurogenetic Diagnoses
The power of hope and the limits of today's medicine
Carole Browner and H. Mabel Preloran

Debating Human Genetics
Contemporary issues in public policy and ethics
Alexandra Plows

Genetically Modified Crops on Trial
Opening up alternative futures of Euro-agriculture
Les Levidow

Creating Conditions
The making and remaking of a genetic syndrome
Katie Featherstone and Paul Atkinson

Forthcoming titles include:

Genetic Testing
Accounts of autonomy, responsiblility and blame
Michael Arribas-Allyon, Srikant Sarangi and Angus Clarke

Scientific, Clinical and Commercial Development of the Stem Cell
From radiobiology to regenerative medicine
Alison Kraft

Barcoding Nature
Claire Waterton, Rebecca Ellis and Brian Wynne

Gender and Genetics
Towards a sociological account of prenatal screening
Kate Reed

Regenerating Bodies
Tissue and cell theraphy in the twenty-first century
Julie Kent

Creating Conditions

The making and remaking of a genetic syndrome

Katie Featherstone and Paul Atkinson

Routledge
Taylor & Francis Group
LONDON AND NEW YORK

First published 2012
by Routledge
2 Park Square, Milton Park, Abingdon, Oxon, OX14 4RN

Simultaneously published in the USA and Canada
by Routledge
711 Third Avenue, New York, NY 10017

Routledge is an imprint of the Taylor & Francis Group, an informa business

British Library Cataloguing in Publication Data
A catalogue record for this book is available from the British Library

Library of Congress Cataloging in Publication Data
Featherstone, Katie.
Creating conditions : the making and re-making of a genetic syndrome / by Katie Featherstone, Paul Atkinson.
p. cm. – (Genetics and society)
Includes bibliographical references and index.
1. Rett syndrome. 2. Genetic disorders. I. Atkinson, Paul, 1947- II. Title.
RJ506.R47F43 2011
616.85'884–dc22
2011004674

ISBN13: 978-0-415-49665-0 hbk
ISBN13: 978-0-203-87815-6 ebk

Typeset in Sabon by Taylor & Francis books

Contents

Acknowledgments

This book and the research on which it is based would not have been possible without the financial and intellectual support of a wide number of people. Our research was made possible by a research grant from The Health Foundation, whose financial support is gratefully acknowledged. The research was undertaken and the book prepared under the auspices of Cesagen, and thus the support of the Economic and Social Research Council (ESRC) is gratefully acknowledged. The work was part of the Programme of the ESRC Research Centre for Economic and Social Aspects of Genomics.

The research is itself part of a much wider series of collaborations between social scientists and biomedical scientists at Cardiff University and we are grateful to the support of colleagues in carrying out this work.

Our greatest debt is to the parents and families who allowed us to interview them in their homes, and to observe their clinical encounters. Social research in this area is not only a matter of cross-disciplinary dialogue between academics in medicine and the social sciences. It is also about the collaboration and support of individuals and their families under the clinical gaze. In addition, we would like to thank the many biomedical scientists and clinicians who have been willing to talk to us about their work and to let us observe their clinical and scientific work at close quarters. We cannot acknowledge them individually, as they have been granted anonymity. However, our research and research like it would simply not be possible if people were not willing to give up their time to talk to us. Last but not least we would like to thank our families for their patience and unstinting support.

1 Multiple sites of a syndrome

In the course of this chapter we introduce one genetic condition – Rett syndrome. Our purpose is to exemplify the main analytic theme of this monograph: the multiple sites and versions in which this medical condition is enacted and represented. We also outline why this rare condition provides us with an analytic window onto wider issues in the sociology and anthropology of medical conditions, notably those with a genetic basis. We begin with a deceptively simple account of Rett syndrome derived from standard medical sources.

The textbook description of Rett syndrome

Rett syndrome (RS or RTT) is a severe neuro-developmental disorder causing profound intellectual and physical disability in girls. First described by Andreas Rett (1966), who published the first English-language account of the syndrome in 1977 as 'Cerebral atrophy with hyperammonaemia' (Rett, 1977), it is characterized by:

> the progressive loss of intellectual functioning, fine and gross motor skills and communicative abilities, deceleration of head growth, and the development of stereotypic hand movements, occurring after a period of normal development. Girls with RS often develop seizures, a disturbed breathing pattern with hyperventilation and periodic apnoea, scoliosis, growth retardation and gait apraxia.
>
> (Weaving *et al.*, 2005: 1)

Rett syndrome accounts for 2–3 per cent of all severe learning disabilities and is potentially associated with 10 per cent of all profound disability identified in girls and young women, with an overall incidence of about 1 in 10–15,000 girls (Clarke, 1996), making this syndrome a common cause of severe learning disabilities affecting girls. Rett syndrome is listed as a rare disease within the USA Office of Rare Diseases within the National Institutes of Health; however, it is above the threshold required for orphan designation by the European Union.

Classically, affected girls are described as developing normally until they reach 6–18 months old when their development appears to slow down. This leads to the start of a period of regression, which may cause a sudden and dramatic loss of skills, although this may have a subtle onset. Regression is often accompanied by social withdrawal, and leads to a loss of skills, particularly speech, with any prior words they have learnt usually permanently lost, and typically they become unable to use their hands purposefully, and girls affected by classic Rett syndrome are profoundly intellectually disabled. Progressive physical problems can also develop in later stages of the syndrome, including scoliosis and behavioural problems. Rett syndrome is not associated with a strong dysmorphic facial 'look'; however, the key physical or behavioural feature is repetitive hand movements that typically develop following the period of regression:

> The hallmark of RS is the intense, sometimes continuous, stereotypic hand movements, which develop after the loss of purposeful hand movements. Patterns consist of tortuous hand wringing, hand washing, clapping, patting, or other more bizarre hand automatisms, during waking hours.
>
> (Weaving *et al.*, 2005: 1)

Rett syndrome continues to be diagnosed clinically based on the observation and adjudication of these key features; however, genetic medicine has also entered the field. A key moment in the trajectory of this entity is the association of a gene with the syndrome. In 1999, Huda Zoghbi's team was the first to link the syndrome to mutations in the MECP2 (methyl-CpG-binding protein 2) gene (Amir *et al.*, 1999). Since then, MECP2 mutation testing has increasingly become available for patients with Rett or suspected Rett syndrome and our local clinic was one of the first to offer this service in the UK. The identification of the mutation associated with the syndrome provided an expectation that the field would be able to identify and fix the diagnosis of children with Rett syndrome at the molecular level, leading to less reliance on the traditional classification based on the assessment and adjudication of clinical features. However, one key obstacle in the use of genetic testing to identify and classify syndromes is that in many cases the clinical and the genetic evidence do not align. The associated genetic change cannot always be identified in children who appear to have all the clinical classic features of the condition, while mutations in the gene are also found in cases who do not have the clinical features associated with the syndrome. We shall follow the attempts locally and within the wider biomedical field to align these two forms of knowledge in more detail later in the book.

Rett syndrome is, therefore, one of a very large number of named syndromes that give rise to developmental delay or regression, and to abnormal physical development in children. The field of research and the clinical study of the diagnosis of such syndromes is referred to as *dysmorphology*. Dysmorphology has been described as 'the study of disordered development' (Harper, 1998: 83) and represents a traditional discipline of delineating disorders affecting the physical development of the individual, before or after birth, and includes the recognition of specific patterns of physical features in patients with a range of problems (Aase, 1990). The specific features that characterize clinical dysmorphology include: the recognition and classification of specific patterns of facial and other physical features; ongoing classification based on clinical diagnosis and examination; and the increasing use and interpretation of molecular tests in diagnosis and clinical classification. Decision-making and assessment of individual cases is distributed and networked between different experts (including scientists and clinicians) locally, and cases can also be reviewed by other experts nationally, and internationally for further adjudication and diagnosis. These features come together to produce variable outcomes, for example the introduction of new clinical categories and diagnostic labels.

The field of dysmorphology is a specialism that displays the interaction of genetic technologies and clinical judgment. We ourselves have already documented some of the devices through which the dysmorphic appearance is constructed, and how genetic syndromes are constituted (Shaw *et al.*, 2003; Featherstone *et al.*, 2004; Latimer *et al.*, 2006; Featherstone *et al.*, 2007). We build on this body of work by following the evolving fashioning and shaping of one genetic syndrome. Rett syndrome was chosen deliberately in order to display the distinctive characteristics of contemporary genetic diagnosis and the adjudication of dysmorphological nosography. Genetic testing had become available for this syndrome and this allowed us to follow the implications of the introduction of this technology as it occurred. Rett syndrome therefore provides us with a snapshot in time, a detailed case study of the effects of genetic knowledge on a syndrome and what it is thought to constitute. This relates back to some of the more general phenomena we have identified in other contexts and for other conditions.

So far, then, the syndrome may be summarized in a simple way. The definition we have already provided corresponds to a 'textbook' form of knowledge. As Ludwik Fleck (1979) first pointed out, textbooks embody just one version of scientific or medical knowledge. Often in summary form, they normally elide features of the condition that are contested, the fuzzy borders of disease classifications or the uncertainties of scientific evidence. They understandably present a somewhat static picture of any given condition, with little sense that the descriptions of conditions – and even their core, defining features – may be subject to change over time. Textbook medicine cannot, of course, reveal the competing interests that can give rise to disputed scientific or clinical definitions; nor can it capture the networks that are mobilized in promoting particular versions of the condition, and the alliances and collaborations that develop. Moreover, the simple, standardized classifications of textbook science do not take account of the practical work that goes into recognizing and describing the condition in a patient. The textbook is equally silent on the multiple interpretations that may be put on a condition by patients or (as in the case of Rett) family members.

In other words, we need to look beneath the surface, or – to change the metaphor – look backstage at the many sites where the syndrome is enacted. We need to follow the condition around several sites and several representations. We need to acknowledge that the relationship between genetic science and clinical medicine may not be perfectly straightforward, and that the identification of the condition may not always be without complication. In doing so we recognize that there are many parties involved, whose interests may vary and whose expert understandings of the syndrome itself may also differ.

Our ethnography traces the syndrome from the local to the international field and back again via families caring for a daughter with Rett syndrome. We follow the work of a local clinical and scientific team within one teaching hospital who were developing expertise in this syndrome. We examine the work within their specialist clinic where cases of Rett syndrome were adjudicated upon by genetic and other clinical specialists (paediatrics, neurology, psychiatry) and their associated biomedical scientific programme (the lead and junior clinician were central to both these projects). It is not uncommon for such teams to have these dual roles; as we have shown, the genetics clinic is an important site for the production and application of biomedical knowledge (cf. Latimer *et al.*, 2006). This group introduced us to the patients and families they saw in their work, and inducted us into the network of biomedical scientists and family networks associated with the syndrome. We traced the syndrome taking this local team as our starting point to map out some of the multiple sites and versions in which this medical condition is enacted and represented.

The spectacular display of hope

We turn our attention to one site where Rett syndrome is assembled and performed. It is based on our observations of international scientific conferences, at which scientists and clinicians, family members and activists come together. These international conferences perform multiple functions, and we shall explore them in greater detail later in the book. They include the graphic performance of different versions of Rett syndrome. These different versions reflect the interests of different professional and lay actors who participate in these international gatherings. Conference sessions shape the ways in which the syndrome is talked about. Particular aspects of the scientific and clinical field are mobilized to promote participants' interests.

At one of the scientific meetings (a Rett syndrome symposia in 2007) we observed, there was an especially powerful enactment of Rett syndrome. Compelling visual evidence was presented in the form of a 'rescue experiment' that was used to dramatize the present and the future of Rett. Monica Coenraads, at that time the head of the RSRF (Rett Syndrome Research Foundation), a US-based parent-led organization that raises money to fund basic biomedical research, gave an extremely polished presentation to the assembled group of scientists and parents. She emphasized the importance of the RSRF and her own role in driving basic biomedical research within the field. Throughout her speech she stressed the importance of developing a cure for Rett syndrome, of reversing its effects. She urged the scientists to take on the challenge. Monica told her audience: 'Since I and five other parents started the RSRF the field has never been the same. There has been an explosive momentum. The principle is reversibility, the possibility of reversibility and translating that to people is monumental, theoretically and scientifically' (Coenraads, 2007). She went on to outline some potential strategies and their proposed 'roadmap' for translation.

This was followed by a spectacular demonstration of the potential for biomedical science to reverse the effects of Rett syndrome. That is, the reversibility of Rett syndrome in a mouse model. Adrian Bird had published this research only a few months previously in *Science* (Guy *et al.*, 2007). In the conference hall, the lights were dimmed. The audience watched a video following an experiment within Adrian Bird's laboratory in Edinburgh. It appeared to demonstrate the reversal of Rett syndrome in mouse models with late-stage disease. The screen showed a tiny brown mouse that looked very sick and was not moving very well around the cage. This was a mouse with blocked MECP2 expression (these mice have an inserted sequence in the MECP2 gene that blocks its expression) and phenotypically it was described as having similar features to children with Rett syndrome. The mouse was shaking uncontrollably and clasping its forepaws, which appeared to mimic the seizures and 'hand wringing' features characteristic of the syndrome, for instance. The next clip showed the same mouse after the team had turned the MECP2 back 'on' (the reactivation of MECP2). It appeared to demonstrate a phenotypic reversal; the mouse had stopped 'hand wringing' and shaking, looked healthy and was behaving like a normal mouse moving around in the cage. This treatment appears to lead to a striking reversal of the advanced neurological symptoms of the syndrome. Bird had only just published this research and it was greeted with loud gasps from the audience, particularly parents who looked very emotional and overwhelmed by what they had seen. The scientists also appeared impressed with Bird's experiment. In this extraordinary atmosphere Monica again stood and addressed the audience with a rousing talk intended to galvanize the group and emphasize its goals:

> I do! I dare hope, I say yes, dare to believe but ACT! We are now in a different situation. Worldwide we are raising fifteen million dollars a year with a particular emphasis on treating Rett.

This set the tone of the meeting. Monica Coenraads and Adrian Bird were the star performers and clearly the leaders of this field. There are close links between them, and Monica's group funds much of Bird's work. Her personal charisma and his dramatic demonstration of reversal in the mouse were powerful enactments of different, complementary, versions of Rett syndrome. Biomedical scientists and family associations come together to create and mobilize a particular vision of the future of this syndrome.

Mobilizing around a cure for Rett syndrome

Following the discovery of the gene associated with the syndrome and its identification as genetic, a large number of groups and organizations have mobilized around the syndrome. While there are many small local and national groups and organizations, the most prominent and successful groups (which act as umbrella organizations and really drive the field) are the Rett Syndrome Research Foundation, the International Rett Syndrome Foundation and the Rett Syndrome Research Trust.

Importantly, the splitting and regrouping of these three key organizations and the changing nature of their affiliations can be closely linked to the scientific milestones and key research findings in the field: the discovery of the MECP2 gene associated with the syndrome (1999) and the reversibility of the syndrome in a mouse model (2007). Each discovery appears to have mobilized groups of parents to increase their efforts to raise money to fund basic biomedical research (at this point the International Rett Syndrome Foundation [IRSF] had awarded US$20 million in grants alone).

Their unified goal – the identification of treatments and a cure to reverse the effects (profound intellectual disabilities) of the syndrome – was boosted by Adrian Bird's rescue experiment. This startling finding quickly became enrolled by these organizations within their fundraising and promotional literature to establish the possibility of a cure for girls with Rett syndrome in the near future. The high-profile biomedical scientists responsible for the key breakthroughs within the field (particularly Bird and Zoghbi) also became increasingly prominent figures in these organizations and on their websites. For example, in prime position on the front page of a fundraising and awareness-raising website is this statement from Adrian Bird promoting this vision:

> We now have proof of concept that Rett syndrome is likely to be a curable disorder. That changes everybody's perception about how to move forward – in a hopeful way.
>
> (www.rettsyndromeawareness.com)

However, the rescue of mouse models has not achieved a similar level of significance for other neurological conditions such as Huntington's disease (Wanga *et al.*, 2005) and Alzheimer's disease (Davis *et al.*, 1998).

This tantalizing possibility of a cure features heavily in the promotion of fundraising activities and these groups variously urge parents via regular email bulletins and newsletters to 'rock for', 'race for' and 'ride for' Rett syndrome. The child with Rett syndrome is also promoted by these associations in a number of key ways and to enhance the broad appeal of the syndrome, sentimental images of the child are produced and reproduced to form a particular construction of the 'Rett girl'.

Promoting the Rett child: silent angels

The promotion of a race to develop a cure or treatment to reverse the effects of the syndrome by these prominent associations has a profound impact on parents caring for a child with the syndrome. It transforms the syndrome from a disorder causing permanent and profound intellectual and physical disabilities into a condition that may be cured and reversed. This adds a further implication that many parents focus on: if the condition can be reversed to unlock their child and enable them to communicate once more, then it may also be a condition that locks in and imprisons their daughter within her body leaving her unable to communicate with the world. This is reflected in the wider on-line community of websites, message boards and email lists, in which it is common to find parents posting comments desperately hoping that a cure is on the horizon for their child:

SUE: Praying some day there will be a cure, I hope that day is soon.
CATHY: Together we will find the cure. The seeds are planted by your efforts, and it sure feels good when family and friends turn out to support, doesn't it?

During a lengthy interview with Annabel, the mother of a young daughter (Charlotte) with Rett syndrome, Featherstone asks her how the syndrome affects her daughter. During the interview we discussed their story from the birth of her five-year-old daughter, when she first started to lose some of her skills (regression), the concerns about her delayed development, the subsequent lengthy search for a diagnosis and receiving the label Rett syndrome for her daughter's problems. Charlotte will always need full-time care and although she can walk, she is unable to feed herself and has no speech. As we talk, Charlotte wanders around the room (her hand wringing and disturbed breathing pattern are both very obvious) occasionally stopping to look at us, and the discussion is tentatively moved on to consider how the syndrome affects her daughter, how it acts on her body. Annabel thinks for a long time and replies:

> Yes, we can feel the effects of the syndrome probably, but whether it actually affects the mind – does she actually know what's going on around her and she just can't tell us, or is it, you know, I think to us we try to think that we hope she can't really understand it all, otherwise that'd be almost like being in prison wouldn't it? I think being trapped in oneself, isn't it? So you've got an expression but you can't express what you actually feel. You can see what's happening but you can't change it or affect it in any way …

Comments such as these from parents suggest one other construction of Rett syndrome. This interprets the affected child as being 'locked in' or 'imprisoned', trapped *within* the body, and potentially able to escape the confines of the syndrome. This imagery is reinforced by the notion that the condition may be reversible. It also reflects the onset of the condition: children appear to develop normally up to a point, and then regress developmentally. This imagery is sometimes developed into that of the 'silent angel'. The image of the 'angel' reflects the appearance of girls with Rett syndrome: they do not have visible facial dysmorphology, and are often physically very small. It is, for instance, telling that the website Rett Syndrome Awareness (www.rettsyndromeawareness.com) is 'dedicated to silent angels everywhere'. It promotes awareness-raising on behalf of Rett syndrome, 'a cause that is near and dear to the hearts of any parent who has the pleasure of raising a Silent Angel with Rett syndrome'. Family associations routinely use 'angel' and 'silent angel' to describe girls with the syndrome. Here, then, is a distinctive 'version' of Rett syndrome that parallels many other conditions. Ways are found to celebrate the attributes of the condition – physical, mental or emotional. Ways are found to celebrate 'special' qualities such as the reported musical abilities of children with Williams syndrome (Sforza *et al.*, 2006), or to *make* them special.

The significance of the MECP2 mutation in labelling Rett syndrome

In the case of Rett syndrome, diagnosis remains a clinical one. Although MECP2 mutations are identified in a large majority of cases, about 25 per cent of girls with classic (clinically defined) Rett syndrome do not have mutations that can be identified by current techniques, and in contrast some individuals with a MECP2 mutation either appear clinically unaffected or have a different set of clinical problems (Weaving *et al.*, 2005). This leads to difficulties in using MECP2 alone as the basis for a diagnosis of Rett syndrome.

Our study also follows the local production of biomedical knowledge on Rett syndrome. The local scientific and clinical research group examining Rett syndrome were attempting to resolving these issues, with a goal to improve the associations between the genetic test results (the genotype) and the physical expression of the syndrome (the phenotype). The team was hopeful that its combined clinical and molecular laboratory work would align these technologies more closely and lead to an improved diagnostic fit. We will follow the work of the local team in collecting cases, searching for new mutations and in aligning its clinical and research findings in more detail later in the book.

In the clinic, physical signs and symptoms and genetic test results are brought together. Sometimes they are aligned relatively unproblematically; however, as we have suggested, the alignment can often prove problematic: genetic mutations can give rise to a wide variation of phenotypes and aligning clinical or behavioural features with a specific genetic basis can prove difficult. The following extract comes from a Rett clinic encounter, in which the consultant geneticist (leading the scientific and clinical research programme) identifies the specific location of the genetic change in a child, describing it as a '1162 to 1172 deletion'. He goes on to say to the parents that it is 'not the most severe' form, but is 'pretty compatible with classic Rett'.

The parents are hopeful that the identification of the location of their daughter's specific mutation will help to clarify her prognosis, her likelihood of retaining some skills, or if she will be severely physically and mentally impaired by this syndrome. However, the clinician emphasizes that there is a huge variation of ability even among children with the same mutation:

> there's a, as you know, a huge range of ability in Rett syndrome and even with children with the same mutation, as there is a huge spectrum of variability.

Here then, the test has little to offer the parent. The child (Georgia) has already received a clinical diagnosis of Rett syndrome and the consultant concludes that even though a specific mutation has been identified, the resulting genetic knowledge 'doesn't seem to be predictive' of the ways in which the syndrome will impact on the child or the likely severity. Genetic testing and other laboratory work do not necessarily align to provide definitive answers for clinicians or parents. Despite their promise, there is not a simple one-to-one correspondence between the site of a genetic anomaly and the physical features of the syndrome. As can be seen in this example, there is a wide range of associated features and the spectrum and severity of the symptoms is variable, a young person or child may have a relatively high level of performance (retain some functional speech), while others may be much more severely impaired.

Adjudicating Rett syndrome

The clinic is an important site in which Rett syndrome is assembled, described and adjudicated. Clinicians may have to decide between competing diagnoses and respond to parents' requests for an unequivocal diagnosis for their child's condition. In the following encounter, a mother and father were attending the clinic with their young son who had previously been diagnosed with Angelman syndrome. Angelman is another genetic condition, first described in 1965 (Angelman, 1965) that gives rise to developmental problems. It is caused by damage to a section of chromosome 15 or a mutation to a single gene, UBE3A. Affected children were originally described as 'puppet-like', and – like children with Rett syndrome – are also sometimes described as 'angels'. The parents had requested an appointment with the clinical team because they had read that some children diagnosed with Angelman were found to have Rett syndrome and they were keen to have mutation testing to clarify his diagnosis:

GENETICIST: I mean, I think some of the children who look as if they have Angelman but have got sort of these Rett type gene changes, some of them have quite a bit of problem with drooling and dribbling and so on.

MOTHER: Oh yes.

GENETICIST: So, I mean, Angelman children can have that so that doesn't really help.

MOTHER: Yes.

FATHER: Well, he's had one of his glands reversed and he's still as bad.

MOTHER: They're on about taking the other one out, just the cold weather it is.

GENETICIST: He's got quite bad eczema.

MOTHER: He's this terrible rash in the cold weather.

FATHER: Yes.

SPR [SPECIALIST REGISTRAR]: And that has been a big problem for him, hasn't it?

MOTHER: Yes, a very big problem. Because he likes going out but it's the cold weather that does it.

GENETICIST: It makes it very sore when it's this cold.

The clinical team and the boy's parents were jointly engaged in a search for the most appropriate diagnostic category. In this particular episode, they all focused on the specific problem of 'drooling and dribbling'. For the parents, this was a classificatory problem, insofar as they were seeking adjudication between the two syndromes, but it was also a practical problem, as the child's face was reported to be permanently wet and sore. For the consultant physician, these features were equally problems for the little boy and his parents, and also an ambiguous clinical sign; this phenotypic feature does not help to distinguish between Rett and Angelman.

The clinic is a site where symptoms and laboratory findings are drawn on in order to classify the individual patient, but to enact the classificatory boundaries between similar syndromes, and so the overall classificatory system of nosography. It is the nature of dysmorphic syndromes that the clinical team often needs to distinguish syndromes carefully from one another; the clinical boundaries between adjacent conditions (often with a range of overlapping features such as drooling and dribbling) are often nebulous and must be adjudicated upon in the practical work of the clinic in aligning specific symptoms within or outside of the classification. In this process there is a major role for expert judgment.

The clinic and the expert gaze

The clinic is not simply a place in which people are fitted into existing diagnostic categories. Rather, the categories themselves are fashioned and refashioned. The clinical encounter involves not merely the assembly of an individual diagnosis. The diagnostic category of Rett syndrome itself is being actively shaped and negotiated amongst experts. By identifying a patient as a candidate for a specific diagnostic category, the clinical team also contributes to the classificatory status of Rett syndrome itself.

A clinical diagnosis and the expertise of the clinician still have the power to fix a classification. Diagnosis is not wholly dependent on the use of laboratory technologies, and clinical perception is not reducible to laboratory findings. In the following extract from a clinical consultation, a family arrives with a young girl with a query Rett syndrome diagnosis. In this context, adjudication and classification of cases takes place between two clinical geneticists (a consultant geneticist and an SpR or trainee) who are leading the local scientific and clinical research group examining Rett syndrome, two consultants from allied specialisms (neurology and psychiatry), and a paediatrician who is a recognized expert in Rett syndrome, known as the 'Rett Queen'. The encounter therefore brings together both the clinical and scientific modes of perception. The following clinical encounter displays something of the oracular pronouncement of the clinical expert. This is an extract from fieldnotes taken at the time by Featherstone:

This is the first clinic and the team all assemble in the children's outpatients unit, based in a new community hospital near the city centre. I meet the consultant clinical geneticist and the SpR who have organized the clinic and they introduce me to the rest of the team, although in this context everyone is introduced by their first name only and no reference to their clinical expertise is made. We arrange the room in anticipation of the attendance of a large number of other professionals working with the family and set out lots of chairs in a semi-circle. Before the family arrives the team chat (quite a few already know each other) and one of the consultants (the paediatrician) reviews the notes with me, telling me about the family and talking me through the child's medical records. Ella is an eight-year-old girl. She is dyspraxic, and regressed at 18 months. She was first seen four years ago. Her head circumference has fallen. She had a viral infection at onset and the paediatrician explains, 'There is often some event that triggers it.' Ella now has no speech, but in the past had a vocabulary of seven words. This paediatrician adds 'classic Rett's' (although they can hear this matter-of-fact statement, none of the other team members respond to this aside). The family arrives and sits down and we all go round in a circle and introduce ourselves. Ella is taken out of her buggy by her mum and throughout the consultation she wanders round the room moving from person to person. She has a pretty, slightly impish face with dark blonde curls. She is dressed in a pretty white cotton top decorated with embroidery, and pink trousers, and she has a red embroidered purse over one shoulder.

GENETICIST: The main thing you were concerned about [he reads from the assessment sheet they filled in prior to attending] were the seizures.

MUM: Yes.

GENETICIST: Is that the main thing?

MUM: I'd like to have the test, I'd like her to have the more detailed MECP2 test. She only had the first one [molecular test]. The literature in the [family association] magazines says you can have the test and find out where the mutation is.

GENETICIST: I have a feeling it's been done. [The SpR flicks through the medical records and they discuss who took the blood and when. The SpR agrees to call the lab to check and leaves the room.]

GENETICIST: So we may have a sample, so we don't need to take another.

The team focuses on the practicalities of retesting. All the other consultants chip in and consider whether the laboratory will need a new sample of blood. However, the paediatrician enters this discussion by stating clearly that this child is 'classic Rett'. Although no one responds directly to this statement, this effectively ends the discussion and the lead consultant geneticist moves on to take a history. He asks questions about the pregnancy and birth, when they first had concerns about her development, whether she had a regression period and what her abilities are now – communication, walking, etc., – and they discuss the genetic test. Once again he is interrupted by the paediatrician who quietly, but deliberately, emphasizes: 'From a clinical point of view she's absolutely classical, we don't need the test.' This intervention puts an end to the rest of the team pursuing that line of enquiry. Interestingly, there is no discussion or negotiation of this pronouncement and the team appears to seamlessly move on to a discussion of the child's 'seizures'. It becomes evident that the paediatrician is the Rett Queen, a nationally and internationally recognized expert in the syndrome. With her embodied expertise of this syndrome she has the power to dismiss the approaches of the other consultants, the molecular technologies and make a definitive diagnosis on the clinical presentation of the child.

The syndrome thus inhabits several discursive spaces. It exists in the clinical and scientific literature; it resides in the personal expertise of clinical specialists; it is to be found in the interpretations of parents and families, and in their negotiations with clinicians. None completely supplants the other. The physician's clinical judgment and expert perception can, as here, take epistemic and professional precedence over laboratory testing. In this particular vignette – and we shall return to this topic later in the book – we also see the significance of highly personalized expertise, whereby select individuals who specialize in a particular disorder can claim privileged perception and diagnostic competence. There arises a sense of almost personal, proprietorial ownership.

Multiples and mobilities

These brief narratives and accounts display some of the facets of a single medical entity – Rett syndrome. We have chosen to begin this monograph with these vignettes and extracts in order to illustrate a key theme. Rett syndrome is a well-established and well-documented medical condition. But it exists in multiple versions and multiple frames of reference. It is produced and reproduced in multiple sites, and through multiple frames of medical, scientific and everyday understanding. Moreover, it has been one of many medical conditions that have been assimilated to the molecular gaze of medical genetics in recent years. In addition to demonstrating the various enactments of one medical condition, Rett also illustrates some key processes in the trajectory of a genetic condition.

In the course of this monograph we shall explore some of these domains of knowledge-production and interpretation. We follow the work of clinicians, scientists, activists, parents and others in the construction of Rett syndrome. This is an especially timely exercise. As one among a vast number of conditions that have been associated with genetic causes, Rett syndrome illustrates some of the most significant developments in contemporary medicine. While the impacts of genetics on contemporary medicine are many and diverse, the identification of conditions as *genetic* is a significant feature of current medical thought and perception.

In following the phenomenon of Rett syndrome, our monograph also touches on the central themes of 'translational' medicine. The theme of translation has assumed a central role in recent biomedical research, healthcare research and scientific policy-formation. It has a number of connotations (Woolf, 2008). On the one hand, the term is used to capture the movement 'from bench to bedside': that is, the development of treatments on the basis of fundamental laboratory research. On the other hand, it can refer to the process whereby research enters into clinical practice, ensuring that research-based medical interventions actually reach patients. The two processes are, of course, complementary. Both refer to a movement *from* research *to* medical practice. As our multi-sited ethnography will illustrate, however, the process of translation is not such a simple and linear process as these elementary characterizations might imply. As we shall see – and as we have already started to illustrate – there are multiple circuits and sites where relationships between research, diagnosis, treatment and social mobilization take place. These are by no means linear processes. Indeed, the processes in question are more complex than being simply two-way influences. The laboratory and the clinic, the family and the support group are all subject to mutual influence. These circuits of 'translation' are multiple, they are just as numerous and diverse as the versions of Rett syndrome themselves. While ours is not directly a study of 'translation' per se, it bears directly on those complex processes that are too often glossed and oversimplified by that rather fashionable term.

THE ETHNOGRAPHY

In order to make sense of the multiples that constitute the various enactments of Rett syndrome, we have consistently tried to 'follow the phenomenon', across various key encounters and institutional contexts. Ours, then, is not a laboratory ethnography, nor is it purely an ethnography of the clinic. Equally, it is not completely dependent on interviews with parents of affected children, although we have certainly included data from such sources. But we have followed Rett elsewhere.

Our original intention – and it remained a guiding research issue – was to trace the changing definition and diagnosis of Rett within the intellectual and institutional context of contemporary medical genetics. We therefore wanted to understand the *trajectory* of a genetic condition. In other words, we wanted to trace how medical genetics had a direct impact on the scientific, clinical and lay understandings of the condition. In order to trace the long-term trajectory of the impact of genetic technologies, fieldwork covered a five-year period. We wanted to explore the meanings of genetic knowledge and decision-making for professionals and families within the context of an evolving genetic diagnostic category.

We have been collaborating with and studying the everyday work of the local clinical genetic service for over ten years. This arose from a series of discussions with a local clinical geneticist about some of the ethical issues genetic technology was introducing into the everyday work of the clinic. Using genetic testing to provide individuals with a diagnosis or their risk of developing an inherited genetic condition has risk implications for members of their wider family. Although the clinical team had a practice of encouraging patients to share this information with family members and to refer them to the clinic, any ethical issues that arose from this fell outside of their expertise. The resulting collaborative study involved Featherstone following the everyday work of this clinical team for 18 months, attending team meetings and consultations across a number of regional clinics, accompanying the specialist nurses on home visits to assess patients and families, as well as talking to individuals and family members who had attended the clinic. The clinical caseload of these regional clinics was highly varied; however, the study focused on cases where a familial condition was implicated, and the resulting monograph concentrates on these aspects of their clinical caseload and the ways in which individuals made sense of genetic risk and its impact on the social relationships of family and kinship (Featherstone *et al.*, 2006).

These clinics also regularly included cases focused on the assessment and classification of children with profound intellectual disabilities thought to be genetic in origin. These cases are usually not familial, but are chromosomal disorders that occur spontaneously (*de novo*) in an individual. The striking feature of these clinical encounters was the close physical inspection of the child's body to look for signs that they might have an underlying genetic disorder or syndrome. Talking to the clinical team we had been initially led to believe that genetic technologies were taking over the field and rapidly entering and transforming the work of diagnosis and classification. Yet despite these technical developments, many genetic abnormalities that entered the clinic could not be identified through the use of either molecular or cytogenic (chromosomal) tests. We were particularly intrigued by the clinical team's use of the more traditional classificatory techniques of inspection and adjudication and the reliance on the expertise of the clinical specialist to 'see' a syndrome; we wanted to follow this work more closely.

This led to an introduction to a specialist clinical geneticist with an expertise in this allied specialism: dysmorphology. This consultant dysmorphologist and her team (two specialist nurses or genetic counsellors) allowed us to follow their work. Featherstone became part of the team, attending their teaching hospital and regional dysmorphology clinics, being part of team meetings and home visits with the specialist nurses. In this service, genetic work is dispersed between consultants of clinical genetics, genetic specialist nurses, other genetic associates, such as genetic counsellors, trainees in clinical genetics (SpRs), other clinicians (GPs and other clinical specialists) and the family. Clinical work is also distributed across different sites: the home visit, the clinical consultation and the regular team meetings.

We found the classificatory system within dysmorphology to be a highly active field in which diagnostic categories are shaped and negotiated amongst experts. At this time a range of molecular tests of varying utility were becoming available – for example, Angelman, Prader–Willi, 22q11 microdeletion and Williams syndromes – and these technologies were starting to be used with an expectation within the field that they would be used to evolve and fix the diagnostic classifications for these clinical categories. It is within these clinics that we first encountered Rett syndrome.

As we were developing this body of work we became increasingly interested in moving beyond the clinic and the family to examine some of the broader themes of classification, the impact of genetic technologies and the wider national and international scientific networks involved in producing and fashioning these clinical entities. We wanted to connect up these local practices of achieving or making a diagnosis, and aligning evidence to the wider scientific networks producing the biomedical and clinical knowledge base; to trace the local, national and international collaborations involved in the fashioning of one syndrome following the production of genetic knowledge and the distribution of a genetic test.

At this time a clinical and scientific study was being planned locally that met these criteria and we hoped to make that our case study. This study brought together a number of our previous collaborators and key informants who were working together to develop local expertise in one specific syndrome: Rett syndrome. The UK expert in Rett syndrome was retiring and was keen for the local team to take over her work; she was handing over her extensive clinical caseload and a UK-wide patient database. The team planned to develop this database by identifying new cases via clinicians who referred cases to their diagnostic laboratory, as well as through their research collaborations. A key part of the process of developing clinical expertise is the collection of a well-classified cohort of types and cases. Importantly, the team were setting up a multidisciplinary specialist Rett clinic where families from all over the UK could be referred. Also, their diagnostic laboratory at that time was the first in the UK to provide MECP2 mutation detection as part of their regular service provision and thus they were starting to receive referrals from all over the UK.

The group also obtained funding to develop their molecular understanding of the syndrome and to study in more detail the cohort of Rett syndrome patients and families who were being referred to them or were already part of the database. Their goal was to improve the associations between the genetic test results (the genotype) and the clinical classification of the syndrome (the phenotype) and to search for new mutations that could be associated with the syndrome. They were searching for new mutations in girls with classic Rett syndrome, particularly in the 25 per cent of cases in which no mutation had been identified, and also in cases where a MECP2 mutation had already been identified. In addition, they were extending their search to look for rare cases of Rett syndrome, such as familial (inherited) cases by examining families where a child with a MECP2 mutation also had a relative with a potentially related phenotype or had clinical or behavioural features associated with the syndrome, such as an intellectual impairment, neurological disability or a psychiatric disorder. The team planned to use this work to develop guidelines for clinicians on the appropriate use of MECP2 mutation testing, and as their grant application put it:

> to develop the most appropriate clinical and laboratory approach to mutation testing in the *MECP2* gene, to clarify the interpretation of test results and to identify the most helpful approach to genetic counselling and testing for families in whom it might be appropriate.

Their long-term goal was to help clinical teams to improve the identification and diagnosis of the syndrome by aligning the clinical features and the genetic findings more closely.

The funding supported the examination of Rett syndrome from a number of perspectives and to employ a clinician (the trainee SpR), a social scientist (Featherstone) and a molecular genetics scientist. This ethnography is partly funded by this grant and it also provided ethnographic access to the wider clinical and scientific research sites. The role of the social scientist within the project was to examine the social consequences of receiving a diagnosis and the implications of having or not a genetic diagnosis. However, taking Rett syndrome as our object of enquiry, we wanted to take this further to examine this entity from a number of different perspectives and sites to explore how this syndrome is created, interpreted and mobilized over time. Importantly, we also wanted to explore what this syndrome means in different contexts and to a range of different 'experts' with scientific, clinical, personal stakes in the syndrome; notably at the local, national and international levels.

These scientific and clinical developments raised a number of issues and specifically we were interested in following the local clinical approaches to diagnostic testing and the interpretation of test results in relation to the evolving nature of the diagnostic categories for this syndrome. This allowed us to explore the interactions between laboratory technologies and diagnostic categories following the discovery of the association between the syndrome and MECP2 mutations. It also gave us the opportunity to examine the hierarchies of expertise, the levels of credibility and evidence and the ways in which differences are resolved among experts. We also wanted to follow the impact of this classificatory work outside of the clinic and into the family domain to examine the experience and impact of diagnosis and how parents made sense of this syndrome and its impact on their child. We also hoped to trace any associated shifts in the diagnostic classification of Rett and its related disorders over this timeframe.

The organization and division of genetic work

It is important here that we describe the everyday work and organization of the clinical genetics service that formed the broader clinical setting for this study. Genetic medicine contains within it a diverse range of specialisms and technologies.

In examining the work of the clinic we do not refer simply to a focus on the core encounter between the practitioner and the patient or 'client'. Nor do we mean we are examining the work of one physical, organizational location within the healthcare system (such as a ward or hospital). Rather, we refer to a wider constellation of settings, clinical staff, and occasions, at which clinicians and others engage in characteristic forms of medical work. Although talking to and examining patients is a key feature, this work also involves examining medical records, and inspecting evidence (such as test results and laboratory values, images and scans), regular professional meetings (such as the clinical case conference), training encounters (such as the clinical lecture or the teaching round) and other meetings with the patient or family (specialist nurses within the service often carry out home visits to initially assess patients and families). In specialist services such as this, what is often called a 'clinic' involves professional discussions that incorporate several of these encounters and layers of work.

We also followed the work of individuals within this network, for example, the work of the SpR in working up cases for both the specialist clinic and the syndrome database. We attended meetings held by the local clinical and scientific team where cases of Rett syndrome were reviewed and where clinical and molecular findings were presented and discussed. In addition, research plans, findings and the management of ongoing collaborations within the field of Rett syndrome were also common themes within these encounters. We also followed the work of the clinic out into the community to conduct interviews with a series of parents who had attended the clinic with their child. However, because of the nature of this condition, the voice of the patient, the child with Rett syndrome, is silent. Observation extended from the local sites to national and international scientific and clinical meetings and conferences, where a large number of informal discussions with parents, biomedical scientists and other experts took place.

The specialist clinic

When dealing with a condition like Rett syndrome, as we shall see, the regular clinics are occasions for teams of specialists to discuss cases and the condition in general, as well as seeing a series of patients and family members. The clinic is a site where the professional authority and experience of clinicians is brought to bear. It is a site at which patients and families are translated into clinical entities.

The specialist Rett clinic was held twice a year and here a range of specialists were brought together – mainly from the local clinical services with a smaller number of other clinicians with specific expertise in Rett syndrome invited from other regions across the UK. Families with a child with Rett syndrome (or suspected Rett syndrome) could be referred or refer themselves from anywhere in the UK. The clinic was based at a paediatric outpatients centre within a recently built local community hospital on the edges of the city. The consultation rooms radiated from a central area, a bright and spacious waiting room with big bins full of toys and dedicated space for children to play, and a number of paediatric clinics shared this space. We followed the work of the clinic over a number of years and the format varied little. Each consultation lasted approximately an hour and the SpR organizing the clinic tried to fit in as many families as possible into each session. This was fairly precarious; families often had to travel long distances to attend, not all families turned up (often addresses and telephone numbers in the file were out of date) and clinical encounters often need longer than the allotted hour. Clinics are unpredictable and cannot be easily predefined as straightforward.

We had planned to audio record these consultations; however, because of the large number of people present and the sensitive nature of the consultations this did not feel appropriate and detailed fieldnotes were taken during and after the consultation. Where possible near-verbatim notes were made, and where we have used such extracts from our field data, this is not intended to convey the impression that these extracts are taken from transcribed recordings.

The clinical team

When a family walk into the clinical consultation, they enter a very busy room crammed with people. The team were led by the consultant clinical geneticist and organized by an SpR specializing in clinical genetics. Two senior clinical specialists attending on a regular basis were a consultant paediatric neurologist and a consultant psychiatrist with a specialism in learning disabilities. Other team members included an occupational therapist and a paediatrician with a national and international reputation for her expertise in Rett syndrome, known as the 'Rett Queen'. In addition, there were usually a number of trainees present and this is where Featherstone was situated with the team. The consultants were all used to being observed by trainees from a range of allied specialisms who were often included in discussions of cases and who were regularly coached in the recognition and management of the syndrome.

When the team introduced themselves to families and patients they used their first names and did not use their titles or indicate their status. For example, the geneticists did not provide their status (one is an SpR and the other a professor, although this may have been implicit in their age and gender) and the paediatrician with expertise in Rett syndrome did not provide any details about her role (although many parents knew of her expertise and were often motivated to attend the clinic because it was an opportunity for their child to be reviewed by her). The clear aim in these introductions was to present a friendly and family-focused clinic.

The large number of clinicians, other experts and trainees present in the clinical team is highly unusual and indicates the unique specialist nature of this clinic and its research focus. In addition, it was quite common within this clinic to also have a large number of experts present as part of the child's team of carers and teachers. For example, one child and her parents were accompanied by their case social worker from the local disabilities team, the child's one-to-one teacher and the head teacher from her school. The atmosphere of the clinic is friendly and it is often a noisy and unpredictable place, children scream, they don't want to be examined, they will not have blood taken and often many people are talking at once.

Leading the consultation

Because there are a number of specialists and senior clinicians involved in this clinic, deciding who would lead each consultation became a delicate process of politeness and deferral. Overall, the senior clinical geneticist acted as the default 'lead'; he had set up these clinics. However, they would usually all lead their own clinics. Thus, prior to each consultation the team discussed the case and agreed who should take the lead in the consultation, usually on the basis of who had prior knowledge of this family.

In this next case, the senior geneticist asks the question and provides the opportunity for someone else to lead. The paediatric neurologist hesitantly offers; she points out that she knows this family and diagnosed the girl with Rett syndrome, but she also acknowledges the expertise of the specialist in the syndrome by indicating that she will open up the consultation for her to take over later in the consultation. To indicate this transfer of status following this polite exchange, she is handed the patient's medical records and moves to sit by the side of the desk:

GENETICIST: Who shall lead on this?

NEUROLOGIST: Shall I do it because I [know the family]?

PSYCHIATRIST: Absolutely, yeah.

NEUROLOGIST: And then I can sort of ask [specialist in Rett] if you would ask a few more questions.

PAEDIATRICIAN: OK. [The consultant geneticist passes her the patient records and the paediatric neurologist sits at the side of the desk. This marks her as 'lead' clinician.]

In later consultations, the more junior colleague (SpR) was given the opportunity to lead. However, this was only where she demonstrated that she knew the patient well by having carried out a home visit and knowing their case files. The key feature that infers lead status is knowledge of the family.

While the clinic opens as a democratic space, it is important to note that the key members of the team with a 'voice' were the geneticist, the neurologist and the paediatrician with expertise in the syndrome (the Rett Queen). The consultant psychiatrist contributed occasionally, but only when there was a specific issue that touched on his specialism. The SpR was sometimes given the space to speak, but only in the context of having met the patient and their family. Similarly, the physiotherapist only commented on her area of expertise: mobility and scoliosis. The SpR and the physiotherapist are also the key team members who played with and focused on the child within the clinic, often commenting on the child and providing reassurance. In contrast, the specialist nurses and trainees remained silent: their job was to watch and learn. The work of interacting and playing with the child was also an implicit part of their role.

The clinic is a site in which professional etiquette and expertise are played out in the collective inspection of patients, the construction of cases, and the production of diagnostic categories. As we shall elaborate in later chapters, the clinic is not a site where biomedical knowledge is passively applied in a mechanistic fashion. The clinic remains a site where medical knowledge is actively reproduced and reproduced. There is no sense in which the innovations in biomedical knowledge have supplanted the practical and interpretive work of the clinician in adjudicating cases and diagnoses. Clinical entities, such as diseases and syndromes, are as much made in the clinic as in the laboratory or in the textbook. The remainder of our monograph will repeatedly explore the multiple intersections of the laboratory and the clinic, the clinic and the family. We shall examine the multiple and shifting grounds of expertise and knowledge that are enacted in these different settings.

2 Making medical entities

> While the focus on illness has allowed sociologists to claim a subject matter, a price was paid for the restriction of a sociological perspective and of ignoring the 'technical' or 'biological' aspects of health care. Sociologists often make a case for studying health and illness holistically rather than with a narrow focus on biological factors but an aversion to taking the 'disease' aspects of medicine into consideration results in gaping analytical holes.
>
> (Timmermans and Haas, 2008: 662)

This observation by Timmermans and Haas is not novel in itself. There has been a consistent lineage of research studies illuminating how technical and biomedical aspects of 'disease' are created and constructed by medical practitioners and others. It is notable, however, for the fact that periodically sociologists seem to find it necessary to reiterate it.

The empirical case study round which this book is constructed is very specific: the definition and recognition of a genetic syndrome. Rett syndrome is an uncommon condition (although it is not universally classified as a rare disease), but it has significance for our sociological interests beyond its medical prevalence. Our interest in this syndrome goes well beyond the specific condition, and we use it to exemplify and explore some issues of much wider significance. In discussing the nature of Rett syndrome, we shall describe some of the ways in which it is identified and defined. We shall explore some of the ways in which it is defined in relation to different criteria and how it is related to other clinical entities in the ever-changing classification of related conditions.

Here, we examine the impact of the MECP2 gene on the classification of the syndrome. The international distribution of a new technology (i.e. the molecular test identifying mutations in MECP2) led to renewed attempts to define Rett syndrome more tightly on the basis of biomedical markers. However, new science and new technologies do not simply appear and transform the ways in which Rett syndrome is identified and delineated. Within this chapter we explore some of the challenges faced by the international clinical and scientific networks in their attempts to develop a stable model of Rett syndrome. We then examine the everyday work of the local clinical team to examine the practical difficulties of managing the variation and instability within the diagnostic category to adjudicate on cases of Rett syndrome.

Creating Rett syndrome

In discussing the nature of Rett syndrome in relation to the implications of new genetic technologies, we describe some of the multiple ways in which it is identified and defined. Rett syndrome resists repeated attempts to fix and stabilize it. Syndromes typically manifest a wide range of features; and this syndrome has a wide range of physical, neurological and behavioural features and a wide clinical spectrum in both severity and morbidity associated with it, from the severely affected classical cases through to a range of associated and milder phenotypes (Webb and Latif, 2001). In addition, the clinical classification of a child may not reflect this spectrum, for example a girl may be classified clinically as having a mild phenotype but has additional behavioural features, which are far more challenging for parents and carers to manage (Colvin *et al.*, 2004).

The identification of a biological marker

As we have already outlined, in 1999, Huda Zoghbi's team was the first to link Rett syndrome to mutations in the MECP2 gene (Amir *et al.*, 1999). This was hailed as the breakthrough in the field that would lead to an improved ability to identify and classify cases of this syndrome, and since then MECP2 mutation testing has become widely available for patients with a clinical diagnosis of Rett or suspected Rett syndrome. The MECP2 gene is located at q28 on the X chromosome and provides instructions for making its protein MeCP2. This protein appears to be essential for the normal function of nerve cells so that they can communicate with each other and is thought to be involved in turning off (silencing or repressing) other genes from producing proteins when they are not needed. So a mutation in this gene leads to a deficiency of this protein, which means neurons in the brain are not able to develop properly. However, the specific mechanism by which MeCP2 leads to Rett syndrome 'remains somewhat of an enigma' (Weaving *et al.*, 2005: 1).

The story of resolution

This point of transition from a purely clinical entity to a genetic condition, with the potential to be defined by a genetic test is a significant step in the career of Rett syndrome. The availability of mutation testing created the potential scenario in which new forms of reductionism could be used to label individual cases in a more objective and standardized way. Insider stories of developments within medicine often imply a process of translation, the progression from ignorance to understanding, from muddle to clarity. There is a characteristic trajectory to the invention of a clinical entity. It often starts, as in this case, with an eponymous discoverer (Rett) who describes the type-case. At a European scientific conference in 2007 an Italian paediatrician gave a paper on the association between the Rett syndrome phenotype and mutations in the MECP2 gene. He provided the audience with a brief historical tour of the syndrome, describing the discovery by our eponymous clinician who first made the connection between different cases, moving on to the subsequent 'struggle' within the field to define the key features of the syndrome. He hailed the identification of the 'MECP2 mutation' as the 'breakthrough' that 'resolved' the classification of the syndrome:

> I am an MD interested in Rett syndrome. I am a relative newcomer to Rett syndrome [...] Andreas Rett observed two children in a waiting room in 1965, then he publishes a paper with 20 patients, naming it Rett. In the 80s and 90s there was a diagnostic dilemma struggling with trying to identify the core symptoms of the syndrome. The breakthrough was Zoghbi and his team [he clearly doesn't realize Zoghbi is a woman] in 1999 when they identified the MECP2 mutation. Since then over 200 mutations have been identified and these mutations account for 70 per cent of classic cases. MECP2 added to the phenotype. This resolved the diagnostic criteria [... He then goes through the key and supportive criteria to a diagnosis and describes the clinical course and stages of the syndrome.]

While relatively new to the field, this speaker demonstrates the wider impacts of these technologies and the hope of simplification they introduce, particularly for non-experts such as this. The story of genetic testing providing resolution is often most seductive to those outside the inner circle of expertise, clinicians whose caseloads may involve seeing only a small number of cases of Rett syndrome in the course of their career. Within the wider field of allied clinical specialisms narratives exist, presenting the identification of the MECP2 gene associated with the syndrome as having resolved this issue of classification.

Lumping and splitting

The trajectories of diseases and syndromes are not so straightforward, however. Soon after the first report linking MECP2 mutations with Rett syndrome, a flurry of studies carried out mutation screening in cohorts of patients in attempts to identify clear phenotype/genotype correlations and define the associations between the biomedical marker and the clinical presentation of Rett syndrome. However, this proved to be not so simple and the results were mixed (Amir *et al.*, 2000; Hoffbuhr *et al.*, 2001; Laccone *et al.*, 2001; Huppke *et al.*, 2002; Weaving *et al.*, 2003; Kammoun *et al.*, 2004; Schanen *et al.*, 2004). These attempts to define the associations between the biomedical marker and the clinical presentation of Rett syndrome are ongoing, as we will see later in the book when we examine the work of the local clinical and scientific team.

The association of the disorder with this mutation, rather than helping to fix the medical classification more tightly on the basis of this biomedical marker, has raised a number of additional issues that have implications for the delineation and subcategorization of this disease entity. Mutations are increasingly being identified in other regions of the MECP2 gene and this appears to be leading to even greater problems of using MECP2 mutations as the basis for a Rett syndrome diagnosis. In addition, other genes associated with Rett syndrome have been identified.

The identification of MECP2 and other associated mutations in genes such as ARX and CDKL5 has led to debates about what subgroups and patient populations are associated with the syndrome and should be included in the classification of Rett syndrome. A number of Rett syndrome 'variants' have been described and these include the 'early-onset seizure' variant associated with CDKL5 (Weaving *et al.*, 2005), the early onset without any apparent phase of normal development followed by regression (congenital variant), through to girls who are mildly affected and a small number who have retained speech (preserved speech variant) (Hagberg, 1989). The clinical criteria were revised in 2002 by the 'Rett Syndrome Clinical Criteria Consensus Panel' to include more of these associated features and other atypical forms of the syndrome (Hagberg *et al.*, 2002).

Other groups of patients thought at one time to lie outside the criteria for classic Rett syndrome are increasingly found to be associated with the mutation. Rett syndrome was initially thought to be extremely rare and always fatal to boys, with those affected by the condition dying soon after birth. However, more recently, MECP2 mutations are now found in approximately 1.3–1.7 per cent of boys with learning disabilities and are associated with a wide spectrum of neurological disorders:

> Today, it is clear that MECP2 mutations in male patients are not rare. Surprisingly, they are responsible for a wide spectrum of neurological disorders, ranging from mild mental retardation (MR) to severe neonatal encephalopathy.
>
> (Villard, 2007: 417)

However, where this group fits within the spectrum of the syndrome is unclear, and raises many questions for the field about whether this group should be included as part of Rett syndrome or whether the phenotype is more distinct and should be considered part of another clinical spectrum:

> The true picture in males is not yet clarified; does a male variant of Rett syndrome exist or is this phenotype lethal and if so why this particular one and not others?
>
> (Webb and Latif, 2001: 219)

Rett syndrome is also classically described as occurring in an individual as a spontaneous (*de novo*) event during the production of gametes (either egg or sperm) and is not an inherited disorder, suggesting it has a low risk of recurrence within families. However, there is an increasing recognition that although rare,

Rett syndrome can be familial. There have been a number of reported cases where there are two affected women within a family (Gill *et al.*, 2003) and locally the scientific team was searching for such rare familial cases. This is of course ongoing and there are continued debates about the syndrome's links with other conditions such as autism, the status of rare variants and the emergence of other allied labels such as 'Rett-like syndrome' and 'MECP2 duplication syndrome' (Ramocki *et al.*, 2010).

Thus, even if a MECP2 mutation is identified in an individual, the interpretation of what this means for the child can be difficult, particularly if a new mutation (in MECP2) has been found and if the child presents with a 'non-classic' clinical phenotype. This leads to increasing difficulties in using the mutation as the basis for a diagnosis of Rett syndrome when there are an increasing number of signs and symptoms associated not only with the syndrome, but with the MECP2 gene itself. There are additional problems in interpreting any mutation identified: how does it relate to Rett syndrome? Should it be part of some other associated condition? Should it be labelled as a rare variant associated with the syndrome? Should the location of the specific genetic change identified be used as the label?

There can be multiple versions of medical knowledge in play at any time with members of the community drawing on a variety of different sources of knowledge, evidence and authority. The range of clinical variation and complexity that genetic technology is revealing, means that the clinical and biomedical field now has to grapple with these discontinuities as it variously attempts to remake and stabilize this clinical entity and align it with the genetic markers.

Creating conditions

Medical conditions are *created* and not merely discovered. More than most phenomena in the domains of natural and medical science, clinical entities – diseases and syndromes – are produced through multiple acts of description, recognition, definition and classification. The categories of clinical medicine are rarely stable. They are always in process of redefinition and reconceptualization. Even longstanding clinical entities that have been described for centuries are subject to repeated definition and description. Conditions repeatedly change.

In describing this as a process through which clinical entities are *created* or *produced*, we in no sense imply that they are not 'real', or that they are conjured up out of thin air by arbitrary or whimsical actions by clinicians or scientists. There is no need – and certainly no evidence – to suggest that medical conditions are not grounded in real phenomena, but the nature of that reality is subject to interpretation. There are no absolute gold standards of reality that are observable independently of interpretation and definition. Consequently, however real we acknowledge underlying causes and processes, that does not mean that we can ever have unmediated perceptions of them. The biological bases of pathology are real in themselves, but they are not available to direct apperception. Consequently, we can never talk about medical entities like diseases and syndromes independently of the systems of knowledge and understanding that frame them, or the classificatory systems within which they are embedded.

At any given time, therefore, we can trace a history, a trajectory or a genealogy for each and every medical entity. These do not have to be traced through a narrative of steady progress. While internalist histories of medicine can be created that imply such a progression from ignorance to understanding, from muddle to clarity, or from belief to science, the record is not like that. The trajectories of diseases and syndromes are often discontinuous. Rather than a smooth series of transitions, we are just as likely to find jerky movements from one set of understandings to another. Major shifts in medical technologies and models at large can create Gestalt switches locally, whereby individual diseases are assimilated to new systems of explanation. Likewise, new systems of explanation create new classificatory systems, creating novel clusterings of diseases, redrawing the boundaries between them, and regrouping them in accordance with new explanatory frameworks.

Creating descriptions and classifications

The history of medical knowledge is marked by changing, often competing, systems of classification. Indeed, the history of medical knowledge itself can be written in terms of its classificatory principles. The branch of medical knowledge known as *nosography* is concerned with the description of disease entities. The principles of classification that underlie such descriptions create the *classes* of phenomena that are grouped together as single entities, and also create the boundaries between different entities.

The descriptions of diseases have their own histories. It would be quite erroneous to assume that the description of diseases and syndromes has become increasingly accurate as medicine has developed over the modern period. For some cases, that might appear to be sustainable, but closer inspection of medicine's past reveals a remarkably varied picture. It would, for instance, seem plausible to assume that pre-modern and early-modern systems of medical thought were founded on classifications and descriptions that have been superseded in succeeding generations. The eighteenth century was – to overgeneralize for the moment – characterized by successive vogues for diagnostic 'systems'. Such systems of medical classification were grounded in a small number of elementary principles. However, such medical systems are barely assimilable to the categories of thought and perception that characterize modern medicine. There is little or no congruence, and one can barely translate between one set of categories and the other.

In contrast, there are descriptions of clinical entities that are entirely congruent with those of modern medicine. The literature of medicine contains many 'classic' descriptions of diseases that may well have been amended and added to, but not discarded altogether. Indeed, the world of contemporary medical knowledge is populated by entities that have a demonstrable continuity with seventeenth- and eighteenth-century clinical descriptions. To that extent, indeed, Foucault (1973) introduced his own analysis of modern medicine's genealogy with a decidedly one-sided picture. He opens his monograph by reproducing two different clinical descriptions of membranes, one taken from an eighteenth-century account and the other from a recognizably modern nineteenth-century account. Both are eyewitness accounts of clinical cases, but appear to inhabit quite different universes of language and perception. They are used to provide a graphic introduction to Foucault's overall thesis concerning the emergence of a distinctively modern clinic and a fault-line in the epistemology of medicine between the pre- and post-revolutionary periods. He stacks the cards in choosing his examples. It is equally possible to include descriptions of diseases and treatments from the later period that are unrecognizable to us today, and familiar clinical descriptions from earlier generations that chime with twentieth- and twenty-first-century perceptions.

If we are to avoid simplistic notions of medical development, then we must acknowledge that grand narratives of smooth evolution are inadequate. So too are narratives of paradigm change that attribute to medicine overarching epistemic styles. As we shall argue, there are multiple, often discontinuous, styles of medical understanding that co-exist, that are intertwined, and that exert complex changes on how disease is understood in general, how diseases are classified, and how individual conditions are described. Foucault's general analysis is thus profoundly limited, although some of his ideas are productive, if used with due care and attention.

Clinical entities – diseases and syndromes – are ideal types. Diseases are constructed out of the symptoms that they contain. Indeed, it is a moot point precisely 'when' a clinical entity 'exists'. The classic descriptions of diseases and syndromes have often been established on the basis of relatively simplistic descriptions and classifications. There is, indeed, a characteristic trajectory to the invention of a clinical entity. The classic description provides the type-case. Subsequent clinical and scientific documentation can render the condition more complex, less stable, more unpredictable and less firmly bounded than the original formulation implied.

To take just one example: von Willebrand's disease is a haematological condition, akin to haemophilia. In a sense, when von Willebrand first described the condition, he was able to do so because he knew *less* about it than successive specialists. It transpires that this condition is highly variable within the same patients, and is even highly variable within closely related kin. The more we know about a condition like this, the less certain becomes the clinical description, the weaker the boundaries that delimit the particular clinical entity, and the more complex becomes the map of related conditions. The identification of a clinical entity, therefore, may involve a degree of simplification. The classic textbook case is often a simplified one, while highly specialist knowledge acknowledges a much greater spectrum of variation and instability.

As Fleck (1979) pointed out in his monograph on medical thought, there are hierarchies and trajectories of knowledge, through which the descriptions of diseases themselves are transformed. At one end of the spectrum Fleck described 'journal science'. This is the textual representation of scientific or medical knowledge in which the potential complexity of knowledge, and the incompleteness of research-based knowledge are represented. The investigative work that goes into knowledge production is, partly at least, visible. There are, however, other domains in which the knowledge is susceptible to processes of *simplification*. 'Textbook knowledge' is one such form of textual representation. Medical textbooks classify and describe medical conditions and preferred treatments in ways that render them accessible to medical students and practitioners. They are, like field guides, handy works of reference, constructing clinical entities in what Fleck refers to as *deictic* terms. There is little or no room for ambiguity and the complexities of journal science are elided. Scientific controversy is replaced with the anonymously authoritative voice of the textbook author. The certainties of the textbook can be distilled yet further, into the yet briefer, pocket-sized vade mecum, lecture-notes or flash cards intended for examination revision.

These textual hierarchies create one dimension of differentiation. They are by no means the whole story, however. If journal science contains some degree of complexity, it is also subject to processes of simplification itself. We know from studies of scientific writing that even journal science is subject to processes of textual simplification (Bazerman, 1981; Myers, 1990). Indeed, the formulaic requirements of the modern science journal paper render some degree of simplification virtually obligatory. The local craft practices of the laboratory are transformed into standardized descriptions, for instance. The logic of the scientific paper is a retrospective, reconstituted account of the study. Positive results are preferred to negative or inconclusive ones. Behind or beyond the paper, therefore, are all of the practical activities that go into crafting research. Behind the written texts of published biomedical science and clinical knowledge, therefore, are the multiple contingencies of mundane incarnate scientific work. The specialist, such as the clinician–researcher, therefore knows – as a matter of professional experience – that the 'realities' of medical entities are more complex and the boundaries more permeable than those conveyed by the standard descriptions of textbook knowledge. Likewise, the everyday practical categories of thought and practice deployed by medical practitioners do not necessarily reflect the complexities that are embodied in laboratory-based medical science.

As a consequence, we need to understand some of the processes of knowledge-production that go into the definition and redefinition of clinical entities. We also need to understand the recontextualization of primary research-based biomedical knowledge into secondary sites of interpretation, such as medical education, textbooks and more popular forms of representation. The diagnostic categories that define clinical entities – and also define 'syndromes without a name' (SWAN) as outside the classification – circulate among networks of experts and practitioners, and between different sites of knowledge-production and reproduction.

The definition and redefinition of Rett

We can see these processes of knowledge production at work in the various attempts by the field in defining and standardizing a number of key clinical features central to a Rett diagnosis. It may be relatively straightforward to classify and record in a standardized way whether a child has normal head circumference at birth and to collect this data at a number of stages in the child's life to establish whether there is a deceleration of head growth in later years. However, standardizing and recording other key clinical features of the syndrome, such as whether the child had a period of 'normal development' during the first six months of life followed by a 'period of regression', is less clear-cut, and is subjective and often based on clinical notes (by other clinicians and non-specialists) and the retrospective stories parents provide, which must be interpreted by other experts later on (sometimes years later) in the career of a particular diagnosis. In Chapter 3 we describe how clinical teams manage and interpret this type of data within the clinical consultation; here we examine the ways in which research groups and the wider field manage subjective measures and transform them into meaningful data that can be used for the purposes of defining and delineating the syndrome.

The syndrome became more widely known in the early 1980s following the publication of the first English-language account (Rett, 1977) and an English-language paper describing a series of cases (Hagberg *et al.*, 1983). An initial cluster of papers went on to describe the clinical features of this syndrome in more detail (Kerr and Stephenson, 1986; Budden, 1986; Naidu *et al.*, 1986; Coleman *et al.*, 1988). Subsequently there were a number of attempts to develop consensus on the key criteria required for a diagnosis of Rett syndrome. The Rett Syndrome Working Group (1988) proposed that a child must display all the following features to receive a clinical diagnosis:

- apparent normal development for the first 6 months of life
- a period of regression occurring at 6 months to 3 years of age leading to a reduction or loss of acquired skills (hand use, speech, communication)
- normal head circumference at birth followed by deceleration of head growth
- develop stereotypic hand movements
- profound developmental delay.

Additional clinical and behavioural features that would support a diagnosis of Rett syndrome include the child displaying breathing irregularities, epilepsy or electroencephalogram (EEG) abnormalities, scoliosis, growth retardation, small cold feet and muscle wasting (Rett Syndrome Diagnostic Criteria Working Group, 1988). A diagnosis of Rett syndrome should be excluded if there was evidence the child had an acquired neurological disorder, a prenatal or postnatal brain injury, eye diseases (retinopathy, cataract or optic atrophy), or a metabolic or neurodegenerative disorder (Hagberg *et al.*, 2002).

Case study: differentiating 'epilepsy' and 'autonomic breathing'

If we examine the alignment of features to this syndrome among the highly specialized leaders in the field, we can see how attempts to differentiate these features within Rett syndrome become more complex and less stable than the original formulation implies. As suggested by these clinical reviews epilepsy, breathing irregularities and EEG abnormalities are all supportive criteria for a diagnosis of Rett syndrome. Defining and classifying these features is an important part of the everyday clinical work of labelling a child with this syndrome. However, differentiating them is often highly problematic for the clinical team. As one of the leading international groups describes it in a clinical review:

> A major challenge in diagnosis may be differentiating seizures from the behavioural patterns often associated with RS. Breathing irregularities such as breath holding and hyperventilation, episodes of motor activity such as twitching, jerking, or trembling, or a cardiac arrhythmia associated with a prolonged QT interval are most commonly confused with seizures.
>
> (Weaving *et al.*, 2005: 1)

This debate could also be found within the international conferences and symposia circuit. A US paediatrician presenting at an international conference in 2005 was in agreement with this approach. He drew on his seniority and expertise in the field to emphasize that such 'behaviours' are not seizures; children with these features (stereotypies, which are repetitive physical movements and jerks; autonomic breathing, which is a serious disturbance in breathing causing hyperventilation and apnoeas) of the syndrome are not experiencing a form of epilepsy, but rather these are features of the syndrome that 'mimic' seizures:

> He starts his presentation by setting out his long-term involvement with Rett syndrome and the large number of cases he sees clinically. He outlines the key 'challenges' of diagnosing Rett syndrome in a child: 'Rett syndrome is not a static disorder, the symptoms change over time and not all children have them all.' He describes the stages and each is accompanied by a slide of a child from his clinic – the first three girls look very pretty and face the camera, the child representing the fourth stage is an older girl with coarser features who appears to be visibly severely disabled. 'I now want to go through some of the challenges that we have with recognizing and understanding Rett syndrome. A key challenge is whether these children have seizures and epilepsy.' He puts a bar chart up showing the differing rates of seizures amongst girls attending his clinic, differentiating between girls who have classic, atypical, and non-Rett syndrome: 'As you can see, girls with classic Rett have high levels of seizures. As you can see, their EEGs are extremely abnormal.' He shows a slide of an EEG with very violent squiggles covering the screen: '100 per cent of the girls have abnormal EEGs and 50–80 per cent are reported to have seizures'. However, he concludes that many of these behaviours are not seizures, they *mimic* seizures [he stridently emphasizes this point to the audience].

In contrast, a different perspective is found at a European scientific conference in 2007 where an Italian neurologist gave a presentation on the clinical features of the syndrome. He too focused on the importance of differentiating whether girls with Rett syndrome have epileptic seizures or other non-epileptic neurological features. His research used EEG and video recordings in an attempt to obtain objective data rather than a reliance on 'parental descriptions' of this phenomenon. However, in contrast to the experts above, he concluded that the apparent non-epileptic stereotypies (repetitive physical movements and jerks) are a form of seizure:

> The screen shows a video of a tiny teenage girl lying on a bed; a tangle of wires are attached to her. The video shows clips of her sitting, resting and sleeping and you can see the irregular and sustained jerks in her muscles. Representations of these movements are then displayed on a graph on the screen. He explains: 'The jerks in the muscle are caused by prolonged delay – cortical reflex – no other condition has this disruptive pattern […] There are huge difficulties to distinguish between seizures and other dystonic movements; few studies have described or looked at this in girls. There is a reliance on parental descriptions, but we used video to understand a girl's history.' The next video clip shows a young girl, all in white, lying on a white sheet, wearing a white head cap with lots of wires leading from it; her body is moving in rhythmic jerks. He ends his presentation with the definitive statement: 'These stereotypies are patterned, purposeless movements and there are usually a range of other conditions when this occurs. There is evidence that they are a form of seizure.'

These expert speakers illustrate the fluid nature of interpretation and the alignment of research evidence and clinical experience that make multiple versions of the syndrome that circulate within and across specialisms, research groups and geographic location, even within the highly specialized circuits of expertise focused on this syndrome. Competing perspectives and the production of clinical and scientific research provide a wide range of definitive statements on one feature of the syndrome, rendering it less stable than the original formulation implied, and multiple forms of the syndrome and its features exist and circulate simultaneously: an important feature of the syndrome can variously be classified as 'seizures', 'epilepsy', 'mimic seizures', 'breathing irregularities', 'autonomic', 'EEG abnormalities' that lie across the borders of the syndrome. The textbook definition does not account for this variation and the complexities and underlying uncertainties in features of the syndrome. Even among experts, we find a process of formulation and reformulation of the clinical entities that constitute Rett syndrome.

The interaction of the clinic and the laboratory to create Rett

There is often a good deal of overlap between 'research' and 'service' in the making of genetic syndromes, particularly in their use of laboratory and other specialist services. Genetic medicine provides us with a clinical domain in which the interaction of the clinic and the laboratory is of fundamental significance. Indeed, it is one of the most interesting features of post-genomic medicine, and it is something that makes a condition like Rett syndrome of special interest. It would be too easy to suggest that there is a simple symbiotic relationship between the clinic and the laboratory, and that the sorts of evidence assembled in the two sites are always complementary. While that may be the case, it is not necessarily so. We have to recognize that the clinic and the laboratory generate not just different information, but different *forms of knowledge*. These modes of knowledge co-exist, but are not necessarily assimilated into a single discourse.

The 'clinic' is not simply a location of medical practice, then. It is also the locus for a distinctive type of medical knowledge. Equally, it is not simply a setting in which medical knowledge is applied. The clinic is, obviously enough, an organizational and discursive space in which medical evidence and professional skills are deployed in a practical way. But clinical work and clinical reasoning go well beyond mere application of knowledge that is produced 'elsewhere'. As we have argued elsewhere (e.g. Atkinson, 1995) the performance of clinical expertise and of professional experience validates knowledge in ways that are independent of laboratory science or of textbook medicine, or indeed of journal science. The clinic represents a relatively autonomous domain of expertise, in which distinctive forms of perception and interpretation are deployed and warranted. Moreover, the clinic is not just a secondary site of medical knowledge. It is a primary location for knowledge-production in its own right. The laboratory, the clinical trial, or even clinical research do not substitute for or supersede the distinctive forms and contents of clinical understanding.

The inspection and measurement of Rett in the child

There is a particular order in working up a case that is adhered to in the Rett clinic. These include a detailed history-taking and the routine detailed physical examinations of the child. In addition, photographs of the face and other unusual or characteristic features are taken (this can include close-ups of the face, eyes, ears, hands and feet, fingers and toes, and spine) and measurements (head circumference, height, weight, curvature of the spine) recorded to show changes in both the individual and the 'look' of the syndrome over time.

History-taking is the starting point for this process. The initial key questions for parents are about the pregnancy and birth, followed by asking when they first noticed 'problems' in their child's development. In most consultations it would be usual to take a history and then begin the physical examination. However, with so many clinicians and experts attending this clinic, the history-taking is not done in isolation and the work of examining the child and collecting the various sets of data occur simultaneously.

It is important to note that while many of the activities involved in the examination of the child are routine for a clinic of this type that focuses on diagnosis and placing the child's features within a named syndrome, there are some technologies employed within this setting that are unusual and not routinely used in general clinics. These clinics include the use of video to record the child to capture the behavioural features of the syndrome and their physical presentation at that consultation. The team record interesting features presented by the child that may be associated with Rett syndrome such as hand movements, walking and gait problems, and breathing irregularities. They record the child variously sitting and walking around the clinic and this type of data forms an integral part of the team's research database on the syndrome, a resource for their biomedical research on the syndrome and an enhancement to their personal expertise.

The team are particularly keen to video Ruby, a rare case, when she attends the clinic with her mother and her grandmother. Ruby has a diagnosis of Rett syndrome but importantly for the team she is considered to be 'high functioning', she has some speech, has the ability to use her hands purposefully and can draw pictures. It is extremely rare to see a girl with Rett syndrome who can speak and communicate. While the consultant geneticist continues taking a history from her mother, the paediatrician (who is a recognized expert in the syndrome) and the SpR take out their small hand-held video cameras and start to record Ruby as she sits next to her mum and ask her if she can walk across the room for them. They comment to the room that she has a 'funny flick' of one foot that kicks out when she walks – this is quite pronounced; they continue recording her movements as the rest of the clinical team stop and watch:

PAEDIATRICIAN: Can you do some things for me first? Ruby, can you do some things for me?

RUBY: Yes.

PAEDIATRICIAN: Will you stand up for me? Now, I just want to see you walking. Can you walk to the door and walk back?

MUM: Walk properly – you don't have to walk slow – walk properly.

SPR: That's better. She's trying hard not to kick.

PAEDIATRICIAN: Yes, she is, isn't she?

SPR: Yes, she really is trying there not to go out. A little wobble.

PAEDIATRICIAN: Very good, well done, that's good. Right Ruby, can you do this one? Yeah that's it, good girl.

The whole team continue to watch Ruby intensely as she walks around the room, and the paediatrician and the SpR continue to video. They are keen to document examples of her speaking, writing her name and drawing for their records and the paediatrician asks Ruby if she can video her while she writes her name and draws a picture of her mother. The paediatrician spends a lot of time working with Ruby, encouraging her to talk to the camera, to draw a picture and to write her name:

PAEDIATRICIAN: Can you tell me what your name is? Pretend I don't know what your name is. What's your name? Why don't you draw me a picture instead?

RUBY: Yeah.
PAEDIATRICIAN: You do that. Can you write your name?
RUBY: Yeah.
PAEDIATRICIAN: You write your name at the top so I know it's yours. OK?
RUBY: OK.
PAEDIATRICIAN: Good girl. Okay, can you draw me a picture of Mummy? [Ruby starts drawing a picture of her mother. It is a very basic stick figure and the paediatrician moves the camera in close to the child to get the details of her drawing action and the drawing itself.]
PAEDIATRICIAN: And some arms? And what about some legs? Good girl. And now can you write mum, M U M at the bottom just so we know who it is; can you do that?
RUBY: Yes.

This is a highly unusual case and is thus highly prized by the team as an addition to their collection of cases and an example of an extremely rare variant within the clinical spectrum of Rett syndrome. Ruby already has the label of Rett syndrome and this is not queried by the team; rather they focus their efforts on recording her abilities (talking and drawing) and the key physical features she displays that are visible behavioural features associated with the syndrome: hand wringing and walking problems. This combination ensures not only that this case is rare, but that others will not query the diagnosis, the visible behavioural features she displays, particularly the hand wringing, verify the diagnosis is Rett.

The team closely record potentially interesting or unusual cases. It is important not only to see an interesting or rare example of the syndrome but also to have collected a case, that is to make a diagnosis and to have detailed records. The images become part of the team's collection and cases such as this can be presented at national or international meetings. Seeing and collecting a number of such rare cases and securing that expertise through presentations and publications can lead to the local, national or international recognition of this team's skill in adjudicating upon difficult diagnostic decisions such as cases on the boundaries of the syndrome.

Collecting cases on the boundaries of the syndrome

A detailed record of interesting cases adds to their database and to their expertise and thus their ability to classify. It also provides the team with the opportunity to test and refine the boundaries of the syndrome and potentially to explore and refine the range of features associated with this entity.

Referrals to this clinic often included families searching for a diagnosis for their child's problems, with Rett syndrome one possibility in many. The focus for the Stein family was to identify the syndrome associated with their son's problems. The team discuss this referral. It is important for this family to have a name; although they have had an initial diagnosis of a different syndrome, this has been queried and Rett syndrome mentioned by other specialists as a possibility. They are seeking a definitive diagnosis for Marcus and have asked for mutation testing. The geneticist reassures them that testing for mutations in the gene associated with Rett syndrome (MECP2) is valuable. In response the parents, particularly the mother, provide reassurance to the clinician that this is what they want, the mother vocally and the father silently nodding. They are both very focused on the clinician during this part of the consultation:

GENETICIST: Let me say a bit about what you wanted to come and talk about.
MUM: Yes.
GENETICIST: Yes, I'm sure it's well worth looking for it [MECP2].
MUM: Good, I was hoping you'd say that.

While a small number of boys have been identified with mutations in MECP2, this is an extremely rare variant (such cases are usually associated with extremely severe disabilities and a high mortality rate). Thus, if Marcus was found to have a mutation associated with Rett syndrome, this would provide the team with an interesting case, potentially lead to a journal publication and would further establish their expertise. More broadly it could potentially contribute to a reconfiguration of the boundaries of Rett syndrome itself – at this time a small number of studies had been published suggesting MECP2 mutations had been found more widely in boys with learning disabilities, and this case could add to that small body of literature. The consultant geneticist describes the association between Rett syndrome and boys, and the level of knowledge at present:

GENETICIST: Yes, no they did think, we did think Rett syndrome was something that just affected girls and in a sense it does, in that, in that, girls with Rett syndrome have this sort of seemingly normal development and then lose skills, yeah. And the boys who have changes in the same gene don't do, they, they don't seem to have the sort of fine development for a while and then lose skills, so they have ...
MUM: To be honest we always said from the beginning ...
GENETICIST: Yes, and we still have, we still really don't know sort of how common Rett syndrome gene problems are in boys. You know, we began to get clues, there were a few boys who had, there were one or two boys who were in families with one or two Rett syndrome girls who were found to have changes in the same gene but a much more severe sort of pattern of problems and ... died, most of them quite young and so we thought they were very exceptional. But then people have been finding other changes, other changes in that gene that don't lead on to death for boys but lead on to something not too dissimilar to the other syndrome.

The clinical team are keen to explore the boundaries of the syndrome and to pursue this chance to identify a novel case or a novel mutation. The consultant discusses the availability of genetic testing and appears to be trying to manage the parents' expectations, indicating that this is available only as a research service and they have a huge backlog of samples to be tested. However, the wait is 6 months, not the 'years' the parents were expecting. The standard test did not find the common genetic mutations associated with Rett syndrome, thus they are now running an 'extension' of the test that is more 'sensitive'. The clinician ends with a statement that it is 'well worth' testing Marcus for this mutation, providing reassurance that they will do it:

GENETICIST: They [the laboratory] haven't found any change in him but there's another, an extension of the test that they can do that's now more sensitive and they want to run it but they're going to have to have his sample. So whether, er ... so that ... I suppose let's hope that one or the other of them at least comes up with things. But I think it's well worth, you know, checking with the Rett gene, yes.

MUM: That's what I wanted to hear.

GENETICIST: But it will take some months ... but within 6 months, or so I was assured a couple of days ago.

MUM: I thought you were going to say years; I did. [Laughs.] [They discuss Marcus' symptoms.]

GENETICIST: How shall I leave it, I mean as soon as I get a result, whether it shows something or not I'll just drop you a note and say we have a result?

MUM: Yes, yes, sounds good to me, yes. [Marcus becomes distressed and they take some time to calm him down.]

The failure in the past to obtain a positive test result does not stop the search for the underlying mutation or gene that may be associated with a child's specific problems. The clinical team often held a strong belief that a genetic change was present within a child and as technology improved, these underlying genetic mutations would increasingly be identified. These parents indicated that they were prepared to wait 'years' for this test and this exemplifies the level of commitment many families have to the clinic and genetic testing in the hope of receiving a definitive name for their child's condition. Here both groups appear to benefit from this encounter: the clinical team have a potentially rare case that lies at the boundaries of the syndrome and the parents are potentially closer to obtaining a definitive name for their child's problems.

In the context of a condition like Rett syndrome, the laboratory is simultaneously a site for the production of routinized knowledge (such as the production of genetic test results) and also the site for the generation of novel research-based knowledge about the condition itself. Here laboratory science and clinical knowledge are harnessed in the interests of fundamental research. This includes research to identify the location and nature of the genetic cause of the syndrome, and to produce a clinical catalogue of examples and variation. The collection of cases has a wider function for the team in terms of expertise and recognition, and having data on a large number of cases provides a store of scientific and clinical capital.

The continual formulation and reformulation of Rett

The more we know about a condition like Rett syndrome, the less certain becomes the clinical description, the weaker the boundaries that delimit this particular clinical entity, and the map of related conditions becomes more complex. The Rett clinic is a site in which some of the messy work of clinical sorting is still observable before its sedimentation in the pure space of nosological systems. As Bowker and Star (2000) make clear, disease entities are identified and defined insofar as they are inserted into broader systems of types and typologies. Such classificatory systems are themselves complex: as Bowker and Star suggest in their discussion of tuberculosis, 'The classification of the disease ... does not stand alone; it is inserted into a shifting terrain of possible classification systems and cultural symbols.' (p. 173). These systems of categories and classifications are, as Bowker and Star suggest, variable. They change over time, and the location of clinical entities within systems of knowledge is subject to change. They also vary in accordance with the division of labour: different systems may be recognized by different specialists, reflecting their specific scientific and clinical allegiances.

In other words, deciding on the appropriate diagnosis and labelling of individual cases does not entail a straightforward application of a predefined set of clinical parameters. As we have seen, in these specialist clinics the meaning of particular signs and features of the syndrome are scrutinized and rather than a debate about the merits of a specific diagnosis, they predominantly focus their attention on where each case fits in the spectrum of features and severity of the syndrome.

Even if there are diagnostic molecular technologies, there are still many areas of dispute in the classification of a syndrome and here clinical expertise comes into play. The classic textbook case is a simplified one. The highly specialist knowledge brought together within this clinic attempts to manage much greater variation and instability within the dynamic category of Rett syndrome.

Case study: adjudication of epilepsy or autonomic breathing (continued)

As we have seen in the earlier section, the scientific and clinical experts within the field continue to debate whether children with Rett syndrome have epilepsy or autonomic breathing (variously referred to as 'epilepsy', 'mimic seizures', 'breathing irregularities', 'autonomic', 'EEG abnormalities'). However, debates within journal science do not assist clinicians in their local mundane practical assessment of whether a child has epilepsy or some other clinical entity. This is a common topic raised within this clinic. Many children with Rett syndrome have been prescribed powerful anti-epileptic treatment and have been diagnosed with epilepsy by other non-specialist clinicians (such as paediatricians and neurologists who are involved in the everyday diagnosis and management of this disorder). For many families attending this clinic, epilepsy is an important, difficult and often frightening everyday feature of the syndrome they have to manage and control on a daily basis. Thus, adjudicating whether a child's breathing irregularities are a form of epilepsy or are autonomic in origin is crucial for the optimum care of the child and often becomes a key focus of debate between the various experts within this clinic.

At any given time, there is not a single medical or clinical orthodoxy in the description of a clinical entity. Definitions of medical phenomena are often variable, and even contested, between orthodox medical practitioners. This should come as no surprise: one of the recurrently documented features of medicine is its degree of segmentation. There are multiple lines of cleavage. Differences between specialisms are one obvious source of variation and in this example we see the convergence of different perspectives on a specific case (or feature of that case). For example, the paediatric neurologist has expertise in the diagnosis and management of epilepsy in children and the paediatrician who is a recognized expert in the syndrome (the Rett Queen) has expertise not only in the classification and management of the syndrome, but importantly in the range and variation of cases that constitute Rett syndrome.

The different perspectives of their specialisms and knowledge of this syndrome are placed in sharp relief when examining cases where epilepsy is the key concern. Isabella is a 16-year-old girl who for many years has been prescribed powerful medication to control epileptic seizures. The lead clinician, in this case the neurologist (who has expertise in epilepsy), takes a history and asks about the 'seizures' and 'odd turns'. The mother refers to her daughter's 'fits' and provides a detailed description of the first episode at age four, which led to the diagnosis of epilepsy:

NEUROLOGIST: OK, to ask you specific things about over the years, has she ever had any seizures or odd, odd turns?

MUM: Yes, I think it was when she was about four years old she had her first major fit. Well, it was her one and only where she turned blue, but up to then she'd been hyperventilating and sort of falling over. It hadn't been diagnosed till then, till she had the fit, and since then she's been pretty well controlled, I mean, she will often, it's hard to know when she hyperventilates whether that is causing her to lose her balance or it is a problem with fits.

NEUROLOGIST: Can you describe what happened? What age that was the very first one?

MUM: The first one was at about 18 months; she did this heavy breathing and her eyes would go wobbly and she, we would have to sit her down somewhere safely and it was more or less dismissed as attention – seeking for a long time.

NEUROLOGIST: So she obviously hyperventilated – it was obvious to you she was hyperventilating – and then to a level where she'd lose, stop breathing basically?

MUM: Erm, never till she went blue; it was just where her eyes would start to roll and she's, you'd have to sit her down or she would just fall down.

NEUROLOGIST: And how often did that tend to happen?

MUM: Oh it was, as I say, it was ten times a day. It was terrible, it was sort of ...

NEUROLOGIST: And that was for quite a long time was it, over two years?
MUM: It was a couple of years; it was when she started school and then she had a major fit and that's when she started on medication.

This description of symptoms is very close to the description of autonomic breathing the Rett expert had provided in a previous clinic. However, the lead clinician and the wider team do not appear to query the diagnosis of epilepsy. Near the end of the consultation, they move back to this issue and the lead consultant says they will write to their GP to recommend an EEG (this test can be used to differentiate the type of event she is experiencing) to provide further evidence. This decision to refer for a further EEG brought the consultation to a close and the mother looked clearly puzzled by this. A referral for this test suggests they were unsure of the diagnosis but this was not made clear and the mother asks whether Isabella should be taking powerful anti-epileptic medication: 'But does she need tablets?'

At this point the paediatrician entered the debate. She called on her status as the Rett Queen to pronounce that this girl may not need to be taking anti-epileptic medication at all and suggested that the EEG results will clarify the diagnosis, which would have to be definitive to warrant continued medication. The mother was clearly not keen on another EEG; it was a difficult procedure and Isabella had to be sedated. The paediatrician reassures her that EEG departments have the expertise to deal with these issues and that a diagnosis of epilepsy should not be based on one event:

> I think any average person would not want to be on medication for one episode that they had at the age of four, and in childhood epilepsy we just don't do that unless you have more evidence to back that up, so I would have thought that trying to get one [an EEG] now would be really helpful.

This changes the whole focus of the clinic and the parents appear astounded at this revelation that their daughter's breathing may be a 'normal' feature of the syndrome rather than something that needs to be highly medicated. The paediatrician displays her expertise by explaining to the parents the underlying mechanism that may be causing this 'way of breathing':

MUM: So this breathing, it could just be breathing, her way of breathing?
PAEDIATRICIAN: Yes, it could very easily be her way of breathing.
MUM: So all these years she's had all this!
PAEDIATRICIAN: I don't know until she's had the tests but I think it could very easily be her way of breathing. I think it could certainly. It's just that the brain doesn't control its breathing or blood pressure or pulse rate well at all so all of these things fluctuate.

We can see the paediatrician display her power as the Rett Queen to adjudicate not only the identification of cases of the syndrome itself but also complex symptoms associated with it. For a feature such as epilepsy, it would be expected that the neurologist would investigate this aspect of the syndrome, and this was reflected (and acknowledged by the rest of the team) in her taking the lead in this consultation. However, the Rett Queen can take over and query this diagnosis. The team change track in light of this pronouncement from their focus on controlling the seizures to using further investigations to establish whether the child has epilepsy or autonomic breathing.

Case study: learning to differentiate between epilepsy and autonomic breathing (continued)

In later clinics we can see the team changing their approach to the diagnosis of this feature to one that builds on, reflects and starts to own the expertise of the specialist in Rett syndrome. We can see this during the following clinic where the clinical team is assembled without the expert in the syndrome. Prior to the arrival of the next case (Grace), the SpR reads the referral letter and summarizes the notes for the team and at this clinic she calls into question the current diagnosis of epilepsy:

SPR: They have a recent positive mutation result. Typical history of Rett, regression and epilepsy. Didn't speak and was initially diagnosed with autism. She is nine years old, and mum has noticed funny episodes of vertigo and breathing changes, but probably autonomic. Apparently she has sleep epilepsy, whatever that may be! I think it's more an autonomic thing.

Grace, a very pretty nine-year-old girl, enters the clinic with her parents and two older brothers. Throughout the consultation she wanders around the room and every time she tries to leave the room (she can walk well) her brothers go after her and gently talk to her and bring her back to their parents. The neurologist leads the consultation and after taking a history the consultation focuses on the epilepsy diagnosis and they study the medical records:

NEUROLOGIST: She has continuous discharges, which can be in Rett but are not always Rett. The telemetries show it's going on all the time.

MUM: Seizures?

NEUROLOGIST: More autonomic. Children can change all the time, it may be coming from the brain, the brain stem, but epilepsy is cortically generated and it's not.

PSYCHIATRIST: It's not an exact science.

NEUROLOGIST: It sounded better in 2001 than in 2000, I don't think it's epilepsy. You've never had a classical diagnosis. It's one of the big conundrums of Rett, what is autonomic and what is cortical. Trying to walk the tightrope of autonomic and epilepsy and whether treatment helps. She does Valsalva breathing [they all study the child].

The team (particularly the neurologist) now appear extremely keen to put their newfound expertise of differentiating the autonomic breathing associated with

Rett syndrome from epilepsy into action. They emphasize to the parents the importance of ensuring the child is not being medicated for epilepsy unnecessarily and to see this as a behavioural feature of the syndrome. Importantly, they also refer to the Rett expert and suggest contacting her about a specific feature this girl is displaying that they have not yet seen in other children:

MUM: Should I be worried about her breathing episodes?

NEUROLOGIST: I think they are autonomic.

DAD: Anything we can do?

NEUROLOGIST: Behavioural interventions, the main point is to keep people from giving her epilepsy treatment [they discuss the child's epilepsy treatment and dosage.]

NEUROLOGIST: That's a tiny dose, it may not be doing much, don't stop the drugs, the autonomic test showed she has continuous activity, just because she may have a seizure if you stop, so keep her on it … clinically, I don't think they are epileptic.

PSYCHIATRIST: Keeping communication, making sure the school knows it's not seizures, they need to be taught to interrupt these, rather than seizures when they are taught not to interrupt, people get scared of seizures.

DAD: So we shouldn't call them seizures, we should be clearer on what they are?

PSYCHIATRIST: Yes.

NEUROLOGIST: We don't have anything to treat these, but behavioural things, give her a cuddle and calm her down, the school need to know that the control of her breathing isn't normal.

DAD: In her sleep she's breathing regularly and slow.

NEUROLOGIST: We don't know all about it. I've not seen a girl with that type of jerkiness before; I probably think we ought to write to [the Rett Queen] to ask her if she knows about it, she knows everything!

SPR: She's seen so many girls with Rett! I'll ask her.

This of course, is not the only point of contention in these specialist clinics. An array of signs and features that may be associated with the syndrome are also scrutinized. Clinicians need to adjudicate whether a period of cognitive regression has occurred; they have to try to derive and agree a description of the child's physical appearance, and whether any particular features are characteristic of the syndrome and therefore of diagnostic value; symptoms such as breathing patterns need to be assimilated into the wider clinical picture of the syndrome, or excluded. Of course, even when the diagnosis of Rett appears unproblematic to the clinicians and scientists involved in the case, this too is an interpretation: the decision has to be made that the facts of the case are indeed straightforward enough to lead to an unequivocal diagnosis.

Conclusion

At any given time, there is not a single medical orthodoxy in the description of Rett syndrome. These are just some of the processes through which multiple versions of Rett and the multiple forms of expertise (scientific and clinical) are brought together to make this entity. New genetic technologies help to effect transformations in the classifications and boundaries of this clinical entity, but Rett is brought into being and made into everyday reality through the acts of description and diagnosis that specialists employ in recognizing and describing its features. Their everyday diagnostic decisions are actively making and re-making this syndrome.

In the course of this chapter, then, we have demonstrated some of the work that goes into the identification of Rett syndrome as a clinical entity. It is important to emphasize at this stage that the production and reproduction of such medical categories sustains the knowledge-system of medicine. It is in this sense that clinical entities such as Rett syndrome are 'socially constructed'. This latter term does *not* mean that they are conjured up wholesale by efforts of imagination or will. To describe a medical condition as socially constructed – or perhaps as we might prefer, socially produced – is to say the following. First, they are not given to immediate perception. Diseases and syndromes do not present themselves self-evidently to researchers or medical practitioners. They depend on acts of description and interpretation. Second, this is accomplished through socially organized work. The clinic, the laboratory and other sites of knowledge-production sustain collaborative work between experts, and between experts and novices, through which the relevant categories of knowledge are initiated and sustained. This depends on a practical engagement with material realities. There is nothing to suggest that clinical entities and the work that goes into them are not real. It also means that the outcomes of this work are not fixed. The separate categories of clinical entities are mutable. Equally – and more significantly – the classificatory systems in which medical conditions are embedded are also fluid. These processes of change reflect multiple processes of interpretation – based in turn on professional and personal loyalties, interests and technological innovations. The fashioning of Rett syndrome illustrates all of these processes.

3 The culture of the clinic

We concentrate here on the spectacular presentation and representation of patients, their bodies and their identities within the specialist clinic. We suggest a broad historical and cultural pattern that brings together the spectacular display and the oracular pronouncement as longstanding (although by no means immutable) features of medical knowledge and the importance of a deeply entrenched visual and oral culture in the creation and transmission of medical knowledge. We trace the intersection of visual culture and nosographic classification in the Rett clinic. The specialist clinic is a site in which we can observe the complex, practical work of diagnosis and of fitting a patient, in this case a child, with Rett syndrome.

We consider this diagnostic work in terms of the spectacular display of the clinic and examine the expert's competence in 'seeing' cases and interpreting visual representations. This is in turn repeated in the expert's right to make 'oracular pronouncements' concerning the patient's characteristic appearance and its clinical significance. We go on to discuss the intersection of genetic technologies and clinical judgment in the identification of this syndrome and examine the other functions of this clinic, the moral and sentimental work of reassurance and of repairing parents' identities in the context of this diagnosis. We affirm the continued significance of the clinic and the importance of resisting premature or oversimplified appeals to geneticization or technologically driven reductionism.

The spectacular presentation of the child

Visual display is a longstanding feature of medical knowledge and there is a long tradition in which patients are translated into reproductions and representations. The medium of photography has provided a rich vein of spectacular representations of individual patients and their characteristics. There have been, of course, many photographic representations of organs and lesions, used to illustrate textbooks and atlases of pathology. The type-case and the classic presentation have been captured through photography from the earliest years of photographic technology and this has been used to compile extensive typologies of characters and social types. Photography provided a mechanical means that complemented and then supplanted fine-art traditions in the representation of physiognomy.

The diagnosis of syndromes relies on the traditional clinical skills of examining the body for signs of underlying pathology. Within general dysmorphology clinics, the photographic image of the individual patient, and the detailed inspection of her or his appearance persists. It can be found in the presentation and discussion of the dysmorphic patient and the adjudication of dysmorphological nosography. In the case of Rett syndrome, the visual culture of clinical medicine associated with this syndrome is significant. Each child is subject to a close and detailed observation by the clinical team during every consultation in order to read and interpret the significance of each feature in the context of the syndrome.

Once the child's history had been taken, the team member leading the consultation typically knelt down in front of the child and initiated the examination by closely scrutinizing each feature of her face and her head (including hair and ears). This examination involved a lot of touching of the child's body by the consultant, using their hands to inspect and feel each feature. The child's hands were also closely examined by looking at both sides and each finger in detail, as were the feet with shoes and socks being taken off. The child was often undressed to her underwear, her limbs examined and her reflexes tested. At this stage the child's back and spine were closely examined for any curvature (scoliosis is a feature of Rett) and the consultant used their hands to feel along the spine, and at this point it was usual for other members of the team to join in and comment on this feature. In this case, they were examining Tamsin, a four-year-old girl attending with her parents, and as the examination drew to a close the consultant announced to the room 'she doesn't have typical Rett feet' (small feet are associated with Rett syndrome). None of the other team members responded to this statement, but it becomes part of the process of establishing whether a feature is within the normal range or a sign of the underlying syndrome. The clinical team were searching in the visual presentation of the child for ways to distinguish physical features, what is normal and what is abnormal, and also which features are part of the syndrome and which should be dismissed. They map the child's body to identify and align it with features associated with this syndrome.

This syndrome has a number of key behavioural features, and thus watching and observing the children within this clinic is important. The clinical team spent a lot of time during each consultation focusing on the child and watching them. In this same consultation all members of the team concentrated on Tamsin, saying 'Hello' to her as she circled the room. This child was very active and walked around the room wringing her hands. All members of the team were very much concentrating on her and on one level this appeared to be a celebration of this child; however, this also had a clinical function: the team were searching for evidence. Typically they were observing her gait, the way she walked and her coordination and also the child's gaze, whether she walked up to individuals, looked at people and focused on their faces. At a later point in the consultation Tamsin was given a biscuit and managed to drop it and spread crumbs all over the floor. This was not treated as a problem that must be cleaned up and managed, but became a focus for the team who all watched her intently, keen to see how she dealt with this incident. Again, this sentimental work also has an underlying clinical function. The clinical team were looking for ways to distinguish her behavioural and physical features, what is normal and what is abnormal. This assessment is based on the clinician's experience of 'seeing' such features and being able to distinguish when a feature or behaviour deviates from the normal range and if it fits within the established features of this syndrome.

Throughout the course of the clinic the team consistently showed their interest in examining any feature in a patient that may add to their knowledge of the spectrum and variability of the syndrome. During the history-taking, the neurologist and the psychiatrist both looked at Tamsin (the same four-year-old little girl) and examined her briefly when she stopped and focused her gaze on the psychiatrist. They whispered together as they examined her and the neurologist took her hand and exclaimed, 'I've never seen that before.' She told the team after the consultation that she was talking about her 'shaky limbs' or muscle spasms, which is a rare and unusual feature, and they discussed whether this feature is associated with the syndrome.

As well as establishing the diagnosis of Rett for these referrals, the team also used these clinics as an opportunity to develop their expertise at seeing this syndrome, and also hoped to see examples of the range and variability of features associated with this syndrome. This will enhance their expertise to adjudicate on cases lying on the borders of the syndrome.

The team discuss Lucy, a 35-year-old woman referred with a diagnosis of Rett syndrome, and on examining her medical records find she has a number of 'interesting' physical features associated with the syndrome that they were keen to see when she attended the clinic: 'It would be useful to see her back, she's also one of the people who has the fourth short toe' (short fourth toes are a feature associated with Rett syndrome and a number of other syndromes). In addition, it is unusual to see women of this age with the syndrome and this case will provide them with the opportunity to see the progression of the syndrome; older women with Rett have different or more pronounced features such as advanced scoliosis and coarser facial features.

The process of knowledge-transmission from consultant to trainee (in this clinic they are all trainees in Rett syndrome) includes ensuring that junior colleagues 'see a syndrome': to see a case within the clinic is also to be able to classify one. The collection of cases and the visual representation of cases (these interesting features are always closely inspected, recorded and photographed) are fundamental to the creation and transmission of medical knowledge (Cartwright, 1995; Kevles, 1997). Seeing a large number of cases of Rett syndrome and establishing expertise by seeing the variability of this syndrome (as well as securing that expertise through presentations and publications) lead to the local, national or international recognition of a clinician's skill to adjudicate upon difficult diagnostic decisions such as cases on the boundaries of a syndrome.

The visual culture of dysmorphology is central. The expert must develop competence in 'seeing' cases and interpreting visual representations. As well as reading the features of the child, the physical features of other family members are examined, discussed and compared. This is part of the process of establishing whether a feature is within the normal range: the team 'read' the child and the parent for visual signs of dysmorphism.

Seeing the syndrome

In this case, the clinician is looking for ways to distinguish physical features and establish what is normal and what is abnormal. This assessment is based on the clinician's experience of 'seeing' such features and being able to distinguish when a feature deviates from the normal range. Here the SpR has assessed a child at home prior to her attendance at the clinic. Jessica, a five-year-old little girl, is tiny and frail (she has a gastrostomy tube); she has no speech and has daily seizures and long screaming fits. As well as taking a history from her mother, and recording the child via photographs and video, the SpR also examined the child's features. During the journey back to the office she describes what she has seen. This child has a number of interesting features and she describes the child's ears and fingers:

> It's quite interesting to see things like her ears. Jessica's ears are sort of … a bit too complicated, a bit too many faults, a few too many creases, the ears are quite long and sort of quite pointy at the top. And then the earlobes are sort of very much attached to the ear but, you know, not connected to the side of the face at all; there's virtually no connection whatsoever between the earlobe and the side of the face so it almost looks like the earlobes are hanging on by a thread … The fingers were really quite short. She had tiny little hands except it was all tiny because of the fingers, the palms were fine, it was just because all the fingers were a bit short and then, you know we talk about clinodactyly (curving in of the little finger towards the thumb), that was quite marked in both hands. It was just these fingers were quite little but it wasn't any one part of the finger was shorter than the rest of it, it was that all the fingers were generally a bit short.

Such features are not examined in isolation but are also compared with those of the child's immediate family – it may be outside the normal range, but a benign feature within this particular kindred. In this case, the child's ears and hands are evaluated and commented on and it is important to establish whether such a feature is familial because if not, it may be a clue to the underlying syndrome.

> I started looking at Jessica initially and thought, oh yes, she's a little bit coarse and a little bit … and a certain something about her that was quite hard to quantify, but you know didn't look, you know, perhaps in the normal range if you like; but then when I was examining her every time I found something, I kept looking at her and then looking across at mum and

> thinking, oh yes, that's mum, so I was looking at her eye shape and thinking, oh her eyes are quite small and quite deep set and so were mum's; and then I looked at her nose and thought, oh, Jessica's nose is quite long and sort of the tip's quite pronounced. And then I looked at mum and thought, well, mum's got a long face, mum's got the long nose as well. She was very much her mother's daughter, you could really see that ... when we were talking to mum that I managed to get a look at her ears and I was trying to get a surreptitious sort of look at mum's ears, now without wanting to make mum feel like I was sussing her out but I'm sure she must have caught me looking at her at times and thinking, 'Oh crumbs, what is she thinking?', but I was just trying to get a general idea.

She explains that while the child's features are associated with Rett, they may also be associated with another syndrome that is similar to Rett: Angelman syndrome. She brings together the features she found most interesting (ears and hands) with her teeth into a general category of bone structure and links this to two other girls with a diagnosis of Rett syndrome she had recently assessed. She lists a number of physical and behavioural features these three girls have in common and whether they fit a diagnosis of Rett or Angelman:

> And you know, bony limbs and short fingers, you know I was thinking well with the teeth, you know is the teeth thing because of something to do with the general bone structure and is that why she's got the delayed dentition? But you know it's all ... but it's just interesting to me that I've seen another family who've got problems with their teeth and unusual shaped teeth, which Jessica didn't have but Jessica did have the gappy teeth and the delayed time for the teeth to come out and delayed loss of her milk teeth and getting her second teeth. And the gappy teeth really made me think of the sisters and then the sisters were both quite floppy, quite loose jointed, quite lax, like Jessica, one of them was particularly coarse, the other one wasn't so much so and they were both a little bit Angelmannian in that they had the laughing.

This child already has a clinical diagnosis of Rett (provided by non-expert clinicians elsewhere), however, this does not mean an end to the search for a definitive diagnosis by this specialist team. The clinician is cautious; the child may just have some features like her mother, but Angelman syndrome was a potential diagnosis when this case first presented and may still be a relevant diagnosis to consider when the family attends the clinic. This SpR is developing her expertise in seeing and adjudicating physical signs as features of underlying pathology and aligning them within the nosography of dysmorphology.

This rhetoric of clinical authority includes the narration of professional 'experience' and in this context the clinician recounts past cases and grounds her knowledge within a biographical warrant. Although this clinician is junior, she has seen a large number of cases of Rett syndrome within her clinical and scientific roles in a relatively short period of time and she directly links a number of past cases and clinical features she has seen together. To have seen a case is to claim direct access to the signs and symptoms of cases and conditions. The phenomenology of the clinic is established by the overriding legitimacy of first-hand testimony.

The collection of types and cases of Rett

The collection of types and cases is an important part of the process of developing expertise. The most prominent visual technology utilized in the process of adjudication and diagnosis of syndromes within the general dysmorphology clinic is the photograph (Featherstone *et al.*, 2004). There are two types of photograph employed by the clinical team, slides taken during the clinical consultation and family photographs. Family photographs are collected at the initial home visit (this is either done by the specialist nurse or genetic counsellor) and are used to examine the child's features, but also other members of the family for signs of an underlying syndrome. However, because most families attending this specialist clinic already have a diagnosis or a query diagnosis of Rett syndrome and because it is rarely familial, it was unusual to see family photographs brought into this specialist clinic. Occasionally family photographs of the child when they were younger were collected and scrutinized by the team, who were often looking for stages in their earlier development when the 'look' of the syndrome could be seen more clearly. Where photographs are available they become part of the evidence used to make a diagnosis and of initiating the process of identifying the child as having a genetic syndrome.

Photographs were taken of every child entering this specialist clinic and they typically featured the front of the face, pictures of each profile and close-ups of feet, hands and any other interesting features the clinician thought may be significant such as toes, fingers or eyes. These slides were filed within the patient's medical records as a visual record of the child and used both to initiate the process of classification and as an ongoing record of their development and changing features.

A number of key features associated with Rett syndrome are behavioural, and video recording of each child was a key aspect of assembling the syndrome within this clinic. Here the SpR was usually in charge of recording the child and cataloguing these cases for the team and their research programme. Recording was usually carried out during the physical examination of the child and continued through the rest of the consultation (as we have seen in the case of Ruby, particularly when there is a rare or unusual case). Video was routinely used to record the overall 'look' and the behavioural features of the child, their stereotypic hand movements, their disturbed breathing pattern. For example, if the child displayed any particularly florid episode of hyperventilation and apnoea during the consultation the team enthusiastically recorded this. In addition, their walking pattern and gait was recorded and any interesting or unusual features, such as the detail of a child's back to demonstrate a particular level of scoliosis. This collection captured examples demonstrating the various stages in the progression of the syndrome and the range of behavioural features associated. It also importantly included examples representing the variability of these features with a focus on the spectacular presentations of extreme or rare variants.

The photographs and video footage can be held within each clinician's own collection of syndromes and features; however, in this clinic they were also added to their research database on Rett syndrome and used as further capital for their collaborative research programme.

Cases used for research and teaching

The collection of cases using photographs, slides and in this case video footage is part of the ongoing process of the assembly of individual cases, but it is also an important part of the ongoing classification and wider delineation of this syndrome. Categories can be refined and the repertoire of 'looks' within the syndrome reassessed by considering this in the context of other clues and diagnostic information identified within the visual representations of these cases.

An important feature of these visual recordings is that other professionals can see them; patients are presented *in absentia* and classification can be carried out without the patient present. They are a form of representation of the patient that can travel to other specialists and can be presented to colleagues locally, nationally and internationally, particularly if a case proves particularly subtle, interesting or difficult to classify. These images are routinely taken to be scrutinized and interrogated for 'clues' elsewhere, most commonly, the local dysmorphology meeting (cf. Shaw *et al.*, 2003), but also at regional, national and international meetings. There is a division of labour among different medical specialties, and there is a hierarchical division of labour among medical practitioners: juniors present the case and seniors adjudicate.

These slides are also collected for teaching purposes; the consultants use them to transmit the process of adjudication and classification to juniors in demonstrating how to see syndromes and read features. We can see this in the transition of one junior, the SpR within the team who had the task of visiting referrals to the Rett clinic to collect detailed case histories, take photographs and video footage and to collect blood samples. Once she had seen a number of cases, she started to demonstrate her new knowledge to the rest of the team. At the start of one clinic the team were waiting for patients; the first appointment should have started at 9 am, and it was 10.30 and still no patients had turned up for their appointments. The SpR was visibly concerned because it was her job to ensure the smooth running of the clinic and she kept checking the reception area, which was shared with a number of other paediatric clinics running that day. She returned to the room and announced that although the family had not reported to the reception, she could see the 'look' of the syndrome in one of the children sitting in the reception area. The door of the clinic remained open and she kept a close eye on people going in and out, saying of one child, 'That's a bit Rett-ish.' She displayed her increasing expertise in this syndrome (this syndrome has a very subtle 'look') in her ability to pronounce on potential cases in the presence of more senior colleagues.

They are also, of course, a form of professional capital and are used for research, journal articles and to enhance expertise and status. These images become part of the clinician's personal collection of types and cases and an important part of the process of developing expertise. They also form part of the team's catalogue of cases within their research programme. In addition, if the case (or syndrome) is particularly 'rare' or interesting, the case can be presented at national or international meetings. At Rett syndrome scientific conferences and symposia it was usual for images of 'the girl with Rett syndrome' to be displayed to delegates via sentimental photographic images and edited video clips celebrating the child and through the presentation of live cases. During the first session within one scientific conference in the USA, a paediatrician with expertise in the syndrome presents a number of his patients – 'girls with Rett syndrome and their parents' – to the assembled audience of biomedical scientists. He has already used PowerPoint to describe the clinical features and stages of the syndrome and, 'Now I want to introduce you to some of the girls.' He shows on the screen a photographic montage of pretty smiling girls aged three to five years old, all wearing pretty party dresses and smiling into the camera. There are a number of families sitting in the front row and he invites them to stand up and 'tell your story'. In response a woman stands up with her daughter, a tiny little girl in a pushchair who looks very frail (she has a gastrostomy tube) and describes her daughter's story to the audience:

> Helen is very sweet, she has a twin. She was diagnosed clinically one year ago and has MECP2. We were shocked, she was a normal child but very delayed in muscle development compared to her twin. We were worried about muscular dystrophy but we were reassured that we had a healthy child – but she was very floppy. On Christmas Eve we thought she had a stroke, she stopped sitting up and using her toys. She's not doing very well, she has a huge number of problems but she smiles all the time!

The presenting clinician adds, 'She's a severe presentation, but she's a cutie!'

There are a number of other parents presenting their child at different stages of the syndrome, a 17-year-old confined to a wheelchair and an 18-year-old girl who can walk. The final mother and father get up with their daughter who is clearly older than the other girls with Rett. The parents each hold one of her hands as they talk about her:

MUM: This is a glimpse of what it's like to live with Rett syndrome. My dream was to have a little girl and it came true, I had Chloe! Rett syndrome affects everything. No one talks about life expectancy and it's like being in the dark. Chloe is 28 years old and pre-Rett syndrome she was able to talk.

DAD: Chloe, give me a kiss! This started our Rett syndrome journey and we appreciate you taking the time to help make a difference.

Chloe walks down the aisle to the end of the auditorium and back and the clinician describes her walking and gait to the assembled audience as examples of classic features of the syndrome.

As we will see later, in the scientific conference a range of technologies and sites are used to see and manipulate the syndrome: in the bodies of patients observed variously in the flesh, via video footage and through photographic representation, and through animal models where versions of the syndrome are also manipulated and produced.

Oracular pronouncements

The spectacular display of the body or its image is paralleled by the oracular pronouncement of the senior clinician. Here we show how clinical authority is displayed through the narration of professional 'experience' and the ability to see and de-code the signs of disease. Medicine has been transmitted from teacher to student through encounters that endure, in form, from generation to generation. The clinical 'round' has provided an encounter in which senior practitioners can demonstrate and expatiate on hospital patients since the earliest years of clinical instruction. The round has provided the opportunity for the junior hospital doctor to present a series of patients to the consulting physician or surgeon since the seventeenth century (this is one respect in which Foucault's periodization of the modern clinic is not universal). The teaching hospital provides a variety of more or less formal occasions in which patients are 'presented' and discussed (Atkinson, 1995). The circuits of discourse display and represent 'cases' throughout the modern teaching hospital. Formal grand rounds are paralleled by teaching rounds in which the explicit function of instructing medical students is foremost.

Clinical consultations also provide the opportunity for the rehearsal of clinical authority. Consultant physicians do not merely display the classic signs and symptoms of diseases and syndromes; they also display their professional authority and status through a number of rhetorical devices. This rhetoric of clinical authority includes the narration of professional 'experience' and in this context the senior clinician has implicit – but powerful – rights to recount past cases and to ground medical knowledge within a biographical warrant. This biographical knowledge is grounded in the warrant of personal witnessing; an experienced clinician can lay claim to a store of first-hand observations. To have seen a case is to claim direct access to the signs and symptoms of cases and conditions. The phenomenology of the clinic is established by the overriding legitimacy of first-hand testimony.

Individual experts in particular conditions can claim – or be granted – particular privilege in pronouncing on conditions that they 'own' by virtue of their special interest, experience or research activities. Experts such as this are also known by families who usually have a detailed knowledge of the field and the key individuals within it, through patient networks, support groups and web forums. Parents often demonstrated their expertise and insider knowledge of the field by stating they had met one of the international experts or that a recognized expert in the syndrome had assessed their child:

> We actually met [UK expert in Rett syndrome] then. And that was interesting, I wanted to meet her because I'd heard tales of her, you know, and we'd filled in a questionnaire for her and sent it off, I wanted to get her opinion.

Syndromes are also named by or after a clinician (for example, Down syndrome) and the clinicians themselves can be named after a syndrome. The wider dysmorphology team within the department occasionally discussed whether to send borderline cases to such experts as the final arbiter of a diagnosis. For example, the 'White Matter Queen' (an expert at interpreting brain anomalies), the 'Angelman Queen' (an expert on Angelman syndrome, a condition which causes severe developmental delay and is characterized by an abnormal gait, characteristic facial features and often inappropriate laughter). Similarly, colleagues may have a local reputation for 'seeing' particular syndromes. For example, during a case review in a general dysmorphology meeting the consultant suggests that they send photographs of the child to a colleague who 'is good at spotting Marfan's'. The opinion of such colleagues is treated with a greater degree of trust; they are often asked to adjudicate on borderline or disputed cases and such classifications are then less likely to be called into question.

The UK expert in the syndrome was attending one of the first Rett clinics; however, it was not initially clear which of the experts in the room held the title of 'Rett Queen'. At the start of this first consultation there was a protracted discussion among the assembled team of six clinicians about the appropriate diagnosis for Ella, with a focus on how to obtain a new and more sensitive genetic test for this child (this consultation was examined in more detail in Chapter 1). It was only when the figure at the back of the room stated 'classic Rett's' that the connection was made. Such a pronouncement that clearly and publicly contradicted (the parents and junior colleagues were present) the diagnostic route being taken by the three other consultants leading that discussion was highly unusual.

The clinician's scrutiny and surveillance of the patient – however cursory or protracted – is endowed with a special significance. The experienced clinician can derive her or his knowledge from a series of sources. The most important is the personal observation of a series of clinical cases. Professional experience, gained through first-hand knowledge, is the touchstone of clinical authority. In practical circumstances of clinical work and talk, such personal knowledge can take precedence over the pronouncements of other experts, the evidence of current biomedical science or the formulations of textbooks. Indeed, the personal knowledge of the experienced clinician – as is the case in many other professional contexts – stands opposed to those who might 'go by the book'.

This does not imply that the expert clinician has no regard for evidence, nor that the claims of biomedical science are completely overlooked. It would be wrong to suggest that they stand in complete contrast. That is clearly not the case. The clinical expert – in this case the Rett expert – is a contributor to the clinical literature, and has a thorough working knowledge of the published journal science in the field. But the specifically *clinical* mode of understanding remains at least under-determined by such public evidence. The clinician's knowledge is not necessarily *tacit*, in the sense that it is often articulated in encounters such as the grand round, the bedside teaching encounter and the clinico-pathological conference. It is, however, *personal*, in that it is grounded in this practitioner's embodied practice and her or his biographically shaped experience.

We can see in this next clinical encounter the ways in which the Rett expert displays her skill in seeing the subtle signs of the syndrome and makes pronouncements on cases. Prior to the consultation, the team examine the notes as they are passed around the room for all to examine and discuss Ruby a 'staggeringly able' girl they have seen before (the first clinical consultation with this family was discussed in Chapter 2). Ruby had already received a clinical diagnosis of Rett syndrome (by the neurologist within the team) and has genetic mutations (in MECP2) associated with this syndrome. The main question for this clinic is why she appears to be losing skills and whether she is experiencing regression or some form of depression and associated emotional problems. The consultant neurologist leads this consultation and focuses on action and treatment, displaying responsibility in her description of her previous working up of this case. In response to the young woman's potential 'depression' she had already referred the girl to a psychiatrist for this, suggesting that she may need anti-depressants. However, after stating her action plan, she quickly deferrs to the paediatrician with expertise in Rett: 'I didn't feel that was within my capabilities.'

The paediatrician immediately changes the focus of their consultation from the discussion of depression as a distinct psychological problem that needs treatment to focus on depression as a sign of Rett syndrome – immediately classifying this as a sign of late regression and asserting that the effects of the regression may be disturbing for this young woman:

> The characteristics of regression seem to be, breathing starts or gets more obvious and that in itself can be very upsetting because with it comes this kind of agitation and confusion. Plus, Why not? Because, you know, the carbon dioxide and oxygen go up and down, blood pressure is up and down, and you can feel faint and goodness knows what else because of everything else […] so I'd be inclined to think that it could be that and so she's having experiences that she didn't have before. So, rather than getting depressed, it's the situation.

The paediatrician also emphasizes the importance of being 'cautious', which could be taken as a mild rebuke to the rest of the team. In contrast to their approach, she focuses on exploring the girl's perspective rather than on the clinical management of a specific symptom. Evoking her years of experience and expertise in the field as the Rett Queen, she powerfully calls on her personal store of past cases to suggest that there may be some other underlying cause and this girl may be in pain but unable to express it:

> And that's another thing but what I would say is, one has always got to be cautious, if a girl is actually distressed, my remote experience, because it's often by phone and they say, well, look for a physical cause and I am impressed with how often a physical cause is found, you know. A woman seems to be doing quite well, and then she starts screaming and slapping for no reason and jumping about and can't stay still and we find she's got gallstones and what have you and it's very difficult in serious ones.

The neurologist brings the consultation to a close, adding that she will write again requesting the appointment with the psychiatrist to treat the young woman's depression. Once more the paediatrician interrupts and changes the focus of the consultation, asking the young woman to describe her experiences; this was the first time anyone had consulted her or asked her to describe her symptoms:

PAEDIATRICIAN: Ruby, could you explain what is wrong?
MUM: Tell the lady what's wrong.
PAEDIATRICIAN: Could you tell me?
RUBY: No.
PAEDIATRICIAN: Can you tell me, do you know what's wrong?
RUBY: No.

The paediatrician once more displays her knowledge as the Rett Queen and reassures the mother that her daughter 'is doing a lot of things which are typical of Rett', giving an account from the young woman's perspective and outlining what the effects of a 'late regression' might be. She implies there is no need for the referral and emphasizes that, based on her expertise, her symptoms will improve:

> I would have thought her sociability and her interest will return. That's what I would expect, not just hope but expect, but her difficulties with movement are so much less than for most people with Rett but nevertheless they are of the same sort. There are movements that interfere and movements that you don't want and there is this sort of tension, agitation, which again is characteristic. I think her body just isn't always do what she wants it to do and that's frustrating. I think you just have to take it as an indication that she needs a bit of space for herself and I think that's the only way to deal with it.

This ends the debate; the Rett Queen has pronounced that this young woman is showing many features 'typical' and 'characteristic' of the syndrome and that she will recover from this late regression in a couple of months. She demonstrates the subtle signs to look for and the importance of focusing on the child. The referral to the psychiatrist is not mentioned again.

Here we can see the dynamic interplay between competing forms of expertise and authority. The paediatric neurologist displayed her responsibility by focusing on the concerns of the mother and by referring Ruby to a psychiatrist. In contrast, the paediatrician repeatedly invoked her experience as the Rett Queen and her ability to see and de-code the underlying signs of this syndrome by linking features of this case to her store of past cases. She re-focused the discussion onto regression and her description of how this may be subtly affecting the child was grounded in her biographical experience of seeing this symptom within other rare cases. Importantly, she powerfully re-focused the consultation onto the child and understanding her experiences. The child's perspective had not been explored within this clinical encounter and was routinely ignored by the rest of this clinical team.

Establishing expertise

At the following clinic six months later, the Rett Queen does not attend and during this consultation, the team display their confidence in having worked up and adjudicated on a number of cases with an expert in this syndrome. Within this clinic they routinely draw on words and phrases used by the Rett Queen and when a point needs to be emphasized, her name is evoked. The family arrive. The mutation testing for Rett syndrome was positive for Camille, a four-year-old little girl; however, their paediatrician had referred them to this clinic because more sensitive testing has become available and her parents wanted to meet the 'experts'. In contrast to the first consultation in this clinic where the team focused on molecular testing of the child to obtain a definitive diagnosis, in this later consultation the team are far more cautious in their approach to establishing the syndrome. Despite establishing a number of features associated with the syndrome, no one appears to be willing to take on the role of pronouncing the diagnosis or state unequivocally that this little girl has Rett syndrome.

The neurologist takes the lead and is non-committal when the mother presents her child's diagnosis (received from a paediatrician elsewhere) as 'typical Rett's'. The mother then moves on to her concern that Camille may have epilepsy. The clinical team exclaims together when her description appears to resemble autonomic breathing rather than epilepsy (we have discussed the assessment of this feature in detail within Chapter 2). Their group satisfaction is similar to solving a difficult puzzle together and they all look at each other in recognition. They discuss Camille's apparent epilepsy diagnosis. The neurologist takes on the voice of the Rett Queen to adjudicate the features of the child's breathing pattern and suggests these 'episodes' were not seizures, but part of the syndrome:

> Her breathing pattern is a bit irregular, which is what you'd expect (in Rett syndrome). Well I think if these episodes are just her shutting down and looking at things, I wouldn't particularly want to treat them.

The consultation seems to drift around the issue of diagnosis, even though this is the key question for the parents and the reason they are attending the clinic. Near the end of the consultation this again comes to the fore; however, the lead clinician does not state equivocally that she has Rett syndrome. Here the SpR intervenes and enthusiastically uses the voice of the Rett Queen to reassure these parents that Camille has a mild version of the syndrome:

SPR: And the only thing she would ever say is that someone who is more mobile now is more likely to be more able later on; so if you're milder at this age you're more likely to be more mild when you get to adult because you're more likely to retain your skills because that's the way that you've been programmed.

DAD: In your opinion then, like, you use the word mild.

SPR: Oh yeah, definitely, because she can walk, she can do hand stretching, she can do things and some people with Rett's can't do anything at all with their hands like she can. In some girls it's really obvious and all of those things are milder.

The SpR uses this opportunity to put into practice what she has learn from seeing the Rett Queen in action, but also her growing expertise obtained by seeing a large number of cases in her home visits. She demonstrates her increasing confidence in being able to place this child within the spectrum of abilities for this syndrome. Here, the diagnostic assessment focuses on the clinical presentation of the child and the positive molecular test result does not enter the debate.

Clinical judgment and genetic technology

The development of new biomedical technologies that can be introduced into the clinic provides the potential for new forms of reductionism to enter into medical knowledge and practice. The identification of Rett syndrome as a genetic condition, and the use of genetic testing to identify mutations associated with this syndrome is a key case in point. The transition from a purely clinical entity to one increasingly enrolling genetic tests is a significant step in the career of Rett syndrome.

However, it is important to establish that there is no simple linear process of geneticization in the identification and diagnosis of this particular syndrome; as we have seen, diagnosis is still made on the basis of establishing the clinical features. Molecular diagnostic tests certainly do not always provide answers that can be treated as unequivocal. First, genetic tests are rarely definitive, so they cannot be used solely as the basis on which to adjudicate cases. In practice, the clinical team moves between its readings of the physical features and interpretations of molecular tests in ways that may well privilege the clinical picture rather than the laboratory-based technology. In addition, even when genetic testing is used, the adequacy of the test may be regarded as insufficient to confirm a clinical diagnosis. However, rather than rejecting the diagnosis, the diagnosis may remain provisional and in this case the child will remain within the clinic.

In consultations with families, the clinical team rarely brought up the issue of genetic testing until after history-taking and the physical examination of the child had been completed. However, parents often appeared quite surprised that genetic testing was not the main focus of the consultation or the key criteria on which to make a diagnosis. During the initial discussion with parents when they attended the clinic it was clear that many parents were attending this specialist clinic in order to gain access to the relatively new genetic test and to have their child tested for mutations in the MECP2 gene. Many described this test as the way to obtain a definitive diagnosis and evidence that their child's condition should be labelled as Rett syndrome. During one consultation the lead clinician (in this case the consultant geneticist) asked the parents of Ella, a child who already had a clinical diagnosis of classic Rett syndrome, why they had asked for this referral and what their main concerns were. The mother replied very forcefully that she would like Ella to have further genetic testing to try to identify her MECP2 status:

> I'd like to have the test, I'd like her to have the more detailed MECP2 test. She only had the first one [molecular test]. The literature in the magazines says you can have the test and find out where the mutation is.

The importance of finding the genetic change causing the child's problems was a focus for many parents and we will examine this in more detail later on.

The centrality of clinical judgment

Although diagnosis of this syndrome is to some extent being reshaped by genetic technologies, in this section we show that clinical judgment is still central. The molecular genetic test does not necessarily enter the clinical process until after the team have reviewed other materials and sometimes they do not enter at all. Even if the syndrome can be identified at a molecular level, the subtleties of the clinical classification are still central to diagnosis. Positive test results can equally be dismissed or enrolled into making a diagnosis, dependent upon the other evidence available and whether it fits with the physical and behavioural signs and clues the clinicians can see in the child.

The subtleties of classification and the clinician's ability to see the syndrome are still of key importance. The paediatrician draws on her powers as the Rett Queen to query the diagnosis of Sophie a 17-year-old girl who had a positive MECP2 genetic test result. She had been given the label of Rett syndrome by her paediatrician (elsewhere) following the genetic test result and displayed some of the key clinical features associated with this syndrome: she has epilepsy, marked scoliosis (onset at three-and-a-half years), hyperventilation and disturbed breathing patterns, but had retained some purposeful hand use. However, the clinical team all noted the absence of a regression phase, which is usually a key feature required for a clinical diagnosis. The psychiatrist leads this consultation and takes a history from the mother (the father is also present) whose key concern is whether Sophie is still at risk of having a period of regression and does this mean she could potentially lose the skills she still has? The team consider this issue and at that point the paediatrician, who has been silent, queries the diagnosis itself, her status as the Rett Queen thrown into doubt by a diagnosis of Rett syndrome without a period of regression:

MOTHER: Looking into the future, do you think she will deteriorate or ...?
PAEDIATRICIAN: Not to answer the question, the question is will there be another mild regression ... if it definitely *is* Rett's?

This is followed by a general examination and observation of Sophie, although crucially no one clarifies the diagnosis. As the lead consultant starts to wrap up the consultation, the parents look extremely puzzled that their daughter's diagnosis has now been called into question. The father asks the team about his daughter's slow response to pain, and in response, the paediatrician displays her authority as the Rett Queen and announces that this feature is 'fairly characteristic' of Rett syndrome and that this feature taken with her breathing pattern and 'temperament' are signs of the syndrome. However, she also calls into question the utility of the genetic test, adding that the identification of a mutation is not a definitive diagnosis because these mutations are also found in a large proportion of cases that are 'atypical' of the syndrome.

PAEDIATRICIAN: Where she's actually been stimulated I suppose, but that's fairly characteristic of Rett. The slow, delayed response to pain is quite characteristic too so I feel a lot of the same things are going on here and it may very well be that there's a problem with the same gene and maybe in a slightly different place where it's just a little bit different. But, erm, with us saying [...] with the breathing there's a lot she's really, she's got a lot of Rett characteristics, yes, but you see they are finding mutations in about 40 per cent, isn't it, of the atypical.
FATHER: Atypical?
PAEDIATRICIAN: So you know they have the same disorder these people but for one reason or another they are just a little bit different so I wouldn't be surprised if you find she has something and it's impacting on the same processes, you know, there's no doubt about that. She's got the same temperament.

Implying that only she as the Rett Queen can see the subtle variation and although the gene may be involved, only she can see and interpret the type, location and impact of the genetic mutation on the phenotypic features of this child. She pronounces that although the girl is not a classic case, she is 'just a little bit different' and places her just inside the borders of a Rett syndrome diagnosis. The expert still has the power to fix a classification and diagnosis is not wholly dependent upon the use of these laboratory technologies, they are still subject to interpretation.

A negative genetic test does not rule out a diagnosis

When the results of a genetic test are negative and the mutation is not found in the child, this does not rule out a diagnosis or a provisional diagnosis of Rett syndrome. The combination of a family actively seeking a diagnosis and the identification of clinical features associated with the syndrome are enough to keep the child within the clinic. The future promise of increasingly sensitive genetic technologies becoming available means that there is always the potential that they may obtain a definitive genetic test result at a later date.

Thus, the team assemble the evidence in ways that suggest that a genetic change is being expressed, even if that particular mutation has not yet been mapped and cannot yet be seen using current molecular testing technology. Blood samples are routinely collected and stored from patients, in the expectation that these technologies will improve and provide families with more accurate or appropriate molecular tests in the near future.

In this consultation, the team report that the recent genetic test was negative in Emily, a seven-year-old girl with a clinical diagnosis of Rett syndrome. However, rather than dismissing the diagnosis the team reassure the parents that the test only provides additional information to the diagnostic process. They will go back and retest using a different genetic technology to look more closely at the gene associated with this syndrome:

MUM: And it was negative when the first one was done?

GENETICIST: But it's just, er, additional information, but sometimes if they're normal then you can then go on to look at the specific gene, you know.

It appeared that if a patient did not fit neatly into a clinical category, this did not mean that he or she was discharged from the clinic. On the contrary, the clinical picture can be assembled in ways that legitimate deferral so that a patient was kept within the specialist clinic. We have also seen that the molecular evidence itself is not necessarily relied on. On the contrary, if there was negative molecular evidence but the team believed the clinical picture of a possible genetic disorder to be strong, a diagnosis was not excluded but would remain provisional.

The team of local senior clinicians assembled for this clinic were from a range of specialisms with no expertise in Rett syndrome itself and at the start of this clinic all were equally focused on genetic testing and providing molecular results within this specialist clinic. As we have seen, it was only after they worked with an expert in this syndrome that they started to rely on their clinical skills to make a diagnosis. Clinicians from other specialisms who may only encounter a small number of potential cases of Rett syndrome during their career, are more likely to rely on mutation testing to provide a definitive diagnosis.

An Italian neurologist described her approach to the diagnosis of Rett syndrome at a scientific conference in 2007. She emphasized that she would never base a diagnosis on clinical features alone and relied on genetic testing as definitive evidence. The following day after hearing talks by some of the leading scientific and clinical figures in the field, she indicated that she planned to change her practice. She planned to re-examine the potential case of Rett syndrome in her caseload 'because it didn't have the MECP2 mutation I didn't diagnose as Rett. ... I will now.' The experts presenting at the conference placed a stronger emphasis on the clinical classification of the syndrome and she expressed a renewed confidence in diagnosing Rett syndrome in cases where no mutation had been found.

Significance of the specific mutation

When parents were provided with the results of a molecular test, they were often provided with the specific location of the mutation if this was available. When the team offered these detailed results to parents they also emphasized the huge variation in the severity and symptoms associated with Rett syndrome and the difficulties of linking the mutation to the presence of specific features or to predict the severity of the syndrome in their child.

The clinical team informed the parents of Georgia that a mutation associated with Rett syndrome had been found in their child and the geneticist read out the specific location of the mutation provided by the letter from the laboratory. However, when the father asked what this meant, the significance of the specific mutation became less clear. The geneticist described the 'huge range' of variability of syndromes and severity within the syndrome in a vague way, adding that the specific mutations do not relate to the severity of the physical features associated with Rett syndrome:

GENETICIST: I think that's true, there are a few sort of trends that people suggest. I think there's a, as you know, a huge range of ability in Rett syndrome and even with children with the same mutation, as there is a huge spectrum of variability. You can say that overall, that some mutations are more mild perhaps than others but beyond that you're only really looking at trends overall. The mutations themselves don't seem to be predictive of what to expect.

DAD: How mild are mild mutations then – it sounds the same question but – yes – I mean how mild can a girl have Rett syndrome clinically but if it is a mild one how disabling might that be?

GENETICIST: Hmm, well, some of the children – it's probably easier to talk in terms of the more, the most mild children with Rett syndrome, people with Rett syndrome – rather than the most mild mutation.

DAD: Right.

It has been suggested that the work of molecular scientists would progressively eliminate clinical judgment and perception in this process of diagnosis and classification, resulting in the 'death of the clinic' (Haraway, 1991). However, the relationship between science and judgment, as is evident in this clinical setting, is not simply a unilinear one; molecular tests neither determine clinical process nor necessarily resolve diagnostic puzzles. Importantly, molecular tests themselves call for more clinical skills and the expertise of the specialist to interpret their findings.

The moral and sentimental repair work of the clinic

As we have seen, the work of assembling a diagnosis is an important function of the clinic. However, it is not the only role of the clinic; other work is carried out within this setting that appears to have a significant function for families. Medical genetics services, like many clinical specialties, are engaged in the production of medical classifications or diagnoses, but also the management of patient identities. Clinical work, is often glossed as 'decision-making', but is embedded in a broader repertoire of moral and sentimental work. The moral and sentimental order of the wider genetic services can be especially significant: the identification of an inherited, genetically based medical condition has potential impact on the social relationships of family and kinship. In specialist clinics such as this Rett clinic where the focus is the diagnosis of a genetic syndrome (this predominantly occurs as a spontaneous event within an individual rather than inherited), this can place in hazard the identity of the child and can also call into question the moral worth of parents. We examine some features of this moral and sentimental work to explore how clinicians and parents co-construct the allocation of moral worth, individual and family identities in the context of these clinical encounters.

The clinical management of children has been a major theme in the sociological analysis of medical institutions and the attribution of identities (cf. Bluebond-Langner, 1978). The intervention of medical services and members of other caring professions in the lives of children and their families gives rise to delicate moral and identity work. The identity and value of the child may be under threat, and may be re-affirmed through interactive face-to-face work; the moral worth of parents may also be a topic of identity work in both professionalized and everyday encounters (cf. Voysey, 1975). As Davis and Strong (1976) point out, the value and attractiveness of children is repeatedly affirmed in the context of paediatric encounters. The maxim 'aren't children wonderful?' (maintained irrespective of their actual performance) captures the taken-for-granted value of children. Likewise, Voysey's analysis of parental accounts in families with a child with disabilities demonstrates vividly the moral work of accounting for 'normal' parenting and 'normal' family life in the face of others' presumptions of family difficulty (Voysey, 1975). Such work has salience for the specialist Rett clinic. As we shall see, the moral order of normal family life and the maintenance of personal identities is a co-production between parents and members of the clinical team.

Blame and personal responsibility was a common theme within the interviews with parents, but was also a common topic they raised within consultations.

Parents frequently voiced their concerns that they might have caused their child's problems in some way and volunteered events or behaviour they felt may be responsible. Being informed that Rett syndrome is a genetic syndrome had a number of impacts on parents' understanding of causation and their role in their child's condition. The potential for identifying the origins of the condition and the potential routes of inheritance provide opportunities for attributing blame and responsibility for the transmission of this condition. Diagnosis also led parents to scrutinize their own behaviour and lifestyle to identify something that may have caused the condition in some way. For many parents, this scrutiny was triggered by their initial referral to the clinical genetic service. For example, once their daughter (Lauren) was diagnosed with Rett syndrome, this was not the end of their search for answers. These parents continued to scrutinize their past behaviour and the pregnancy to find a possible cause and consider whether they had 'done something' to cause or trigger the onset of Lauren's problems:

KATE: You actually feel so guilty because it could have been something you did to affect her. You think, what did we do? Did we give her this wrong? or did we do something at the time? or, you know. We used to question it every day. Everything has got to be done for her. So it is a shock and you think to yourself, you know, how did this actually happen? I used to think it was the whooping cough.

MARK: As I said, when she [his wife] was feeling guilty, I was thinking it was my fault. This goes through our minds all the time.

An important aspect of these clinical consultations was the work of repairing the perceptions of identity of the child and the family. Attendance at the clinic meant that parents were in an environment where their child was routinely admired by the clinical team, rather than treated as a potential source of shame and stigma. Although this clinic was in the context of identifying a condition with potentially dysmorphic or physically apparent features, the clinical team routinely described the child in terms of their physical attractiveness. It was usual for them to describe each child variously as 'delightful', 'gorgeous', 'beautiful', 'a delight', 'captivating'.

The clinical team spent a large proportion of each consultation focusing on the child. Although this was predominantly to assess the child and to identify physical and behavioural features of the syndrome, it also served to make the child special and provided an opportunity to celebrate their abilities. After the initial consultation the Alford family were led to a side room for a second consultation to examine Rosie's scoliosis, a key problem for children with Rett syndrome. Whilst this part of the consultation focused on mobility and preventing further curvature of the spine, it also included a lot of praise for the child, the parents and their team of carers. They were provided with reassurance that they were doing the right things for their child and were exemplary in their care. Both parents radiated pride as they were praised for presenting the clinical team with a girl who was a 'delight to see':

[We all move to a smaller consultation room dominated by the examination table. The physiotherapist sits next to her desk, which is dominated by clinical models of vertebrae and joints.]

PHYSIOTHERAPIST: Older girls all have it [scoliosis] so you have to do everything you can to help prevent this.

[The child wanders around the room and everyone watches her.]

PHYSIOTHERAPIST: Good feet, walking tall, shoulders slightly forwards, probably because she's using her hands a lot.

[She examines her on the table, she rotates her shoulder and suggests the parents do it regularly to ensure she continues to have the full range of movement. She lays the child on her front and shows the mother exercises to do to keep her back straight.]

PHYSIOTHERAPIST: That's me done, she's a delight to see!

These clinical encounters were also an opportunity for parents to take pride in their child, and to demonstrate they were a 'normal' family. It was common for parents to tell the clinical team they were 'lucky' to have their child and that they 'try to live every day as normal'. These parents actively demonstrated this to the team: this mother described their luck in having such a child, but also implied this was because of the work they put in to look after her, while her husband focused on Rosie, adjusting her clothes and putting her bag neatly on her shoulder, a demonstration of the care they take in looking after her. Rosie was dressed in fashionable clothes typical for that age group, in jeans embroidered with flowers and a pastel sweatshirt:

MUM: I think at the end of the day it's how you are with them, we're very lucky and that's why she is as she is.
PHYSIOTHERAPIST: She still has the ability to learn, if you expect low results you get low results.
MUM: I try to live every day as normal.

Presenting themselves as good parents, being a normal family and having a normal child was an unspoken but clear goal of all the families attending this clinic. Almost every girl attending the clinic was dressed with care and attention in the latest clothes for her age group in pinks and pastel colours, with bags, and accessories, all beautifully groomed and hair often elaborately styled.

Reassurance and expertise

The clinical team routinely reassured parents that they were doing the best for their child and praised them for being good parents. The pursuit of a genetic diagnosis provides parents with an extended consultation with an expert on their child's condition. In these specialist clinics it would be normal to have a one-hour appointment, and some last for two hours or more; not so with other specialisms. The child's development was monitored and assessed over an extended period during which a number of investigations are carried out, usually over a number of years. In turn, parents often reassured the clinical team about the benefits of attending the clinic, the development of the child and their ability to cope with their child's disabilities.

The severity of each child's condition was usually explicitly placed within the scale and severity of the spectrum of problems associated with Rett syndrome. The clinical team often reassured parents that their child had a mild form of the syndrome or was developing better than expected. Clinicians display their expertise by locating the child's condition within their own biographical frame of reference. Because they have seen a large number of children with this rare condition, they are able to comment authoritatively on the child's prognosis and where they are on the spectrum of severity for this syndrome. However, although the clinical team may place children at the severe end of the spectrum, it would be unusual to see a child classified and explicitly presented as such to parents.

The clinic also functions as a confessional space; parents discuss their fears and concerns about their children. In the second consultation with Ruby and her mother, the Rett expert provides the mother with definitive reassurance about her daughter's development and progress. Ruby is mildly affected by Rett syndrome and has good communication skills; however, her mother tells the clinical team that her greatest fear is that her daughter may lose 'everything literally overnight'. The paediatrician provides reassurance by calling on her biographical warrant as the Rett Queen: she has never seen a case where this has happened. She concludes that Ruby is 'doing well'; a 'lovely girl' who has 'concrete thought':

MUM: I have given up years ago thinking we are going to get a magic pill, you know, that will make it all … but it just sort of … I think the biggest fear that I've got is one day I am going to wake up and we have lost everything. Literally overnight. I know nobody can say that no, that's not going to happen – because I don't suppose anybody knows.

PAEDIATRICIAN: I haven't seen it happen and that's something.

MUM: But knowing my luck she would be the one in a million that it would happen to because she's always been the one in a million that have got it.

PAEDIATRICIAN: There are a few others who … In fact, what I should do is send you a copy of the paper put together with the help of her grandmother and a girl who is able, and that was very interesting because, in fact, the girl herself was able to write some of her own ideas and so on and she has done very well. I think this will be the general experience and I think this is quite a consistent experience that people who are doing as well as Ruby go on doing well. So during this time it's more a matter of being supportive, making room for her and almost as if she was having something like a

> migraine or a fit. Which she probably is not but in the same way you just give her personal space, you know; they're having a difficult time and it's not their fault and see if the situation ... She is a lovely girl and she seems to have concrete thought with this conversation about the dress you got and where you got it, you know.

This suggests that ongoing contact with the genetics clinic serves to provide a wider role than simply that of providing a diagnosis. It is a role that parents value. Although obtaining a diagnosis can be very important to families, such contact beyond diagnosis can provide important support for the parents and may well be in direct contrast to the attitudes they encounter in other areas of their life.

Conclusion

In the course of this chapter we have followed Rett syndrome into the clinic. We have emphasized a number of related issues. Throughout, we have stressed the fact that the clinic retains its centrality and its distinctiveness even in the context of geneticized medicine.

It has been too easy for sociologists and other observers to claim or to imply that the clinic is of reduced significance in a world of technologically driven biomedicine. It is tempting, and indeed fashionable, to classify the history of medical knowledge in terms of distinct periods, and to attach distinctive modes of knowledge-production to them in turn. On that basis, we might expect laboratory-led developments such as genetic testing to have superseded 'clinical' modes of perception and inference. That is not the case.

As we have seen, the clinic retains its significance within the culture of hospital medicine. It remains a site for the display and inspection of patients, and for their transformation into 'cases'. In this clinical mode of work, the senior clinician continues to enact her or his personal knowledge. Clinical expertise is legitimated in various ways. They include appeals to scientifically based clinical or fundamental research. But they also include appeals to personal authority. The clinical perception and interpretation of the manifestations of medical entities is not reducible to the enumeration of laboratory values, test results and the like.

Moreover, as we have also seen, the boundaries between clinical entities are not hard-and-fast. The experienced clinician retains the right to discriminate. The competence to create fine distinctions, and so to distinguish between similar syndromes and other conditions, is central to clinical expertise. Again, this is not coterminous with the results of laboratory tests, such as those of the new medical genetics. Equally, the clinician claims the expertise to judge whether a feature is diagnostically relevant or incidental to the case in hand.

While we do not wish to imply that expert clinicians are wilfully oblivious of other sources of evidence and legitimation, we do wish to emphasize that within the clinic – as a discursive space – there co-exist multiple sources of knowledge and legitimation. Consequently, rather than thinking of successive phases or stages of medical knowledge, and emphasizing the discontinuities between them, we need equally to recognize that there are multiple forms of knowledge in play in the clinic. Rather than identifying a succession of types of medical knowledge, we prefer to think of the clinic as a palimpsest, in which the *longue durée* of clinical understanding intersects with more recent forms of biomedical understanding.

Genetic conditions like Rett syndrome are especially relevant to our general understanding of this phenomenon. We have already seen that molecular biology and the development of genetic testing have *not* resulted in a simplified, reductionist version of the condition. The identification of a genetic basis does not remove all ambiguity concerning the classification and description of the disease. The medicine of signs and symptoms is not reduced to a medicine of laboratory tests. Consequently, as we have attempted to show in this chapter, the clinic retains its significance in the enactment of medical entities. The clinical mentality and the distinctive forms of clinical reasoning have a remarkable resilience. They too are not reduced to the routine application of laboratory-derived evidence.

4 The transformation of patienthood

Accounts of the transformation of clinical medicine are also linked to narratives concerning the medical construction of patienthood. Just as the trajectories of technoscientific change imply a transformed – often reduced – medical practitioner, so too they imply a transformation in patienthood. Rett syndrome provides an opportunity for us to examine some of the consequences of genetic medicine for patients and family members.

The patient in contemporary, biomedicalized medicine is portrayed primarily in terms of a constellation of factors that help construct new kinds of biomedical identities. They include an emphasis on risk rather than overt disease, the imperative for people to act as responsible consumers of health care, and to be morally responsible for their own care (cf. Clarke *et al.*, 2003). It is also argued that this version of patienthood reflects a more general neoliberal ideology, with an emphasis on individual responsibility, self-management and choice. From this perspective, the gaze of medicine is no longer directed at the patient but on the population, and of the non-symptomatic individual, through an imperative of self-surveillance on the part of responsible individuals, through the identification of risk factors and values, and through the endorsement of health-promoting regimes. Biological citizenship thus rests on new forms of governmentality, it is claimed, that include transformations in personal identity, under the widened gaze of organized medicine.

These transformations in turn imply not only individual responsibility, but also newly emergent phenomena such as 'biological citizenship' (e.g. Rose, 2006). Its proponents argue that biological citizenship arises through the construction of individual and collective identities through biological or medical categories. The transformations of medicine that give rise to its molecularization and geneticization are central to this process of reconfiguration. The rise of genetic medicine in particular is held to produce key transformations in patienthood, and indeed in personhood. We have already made reference to the 'geneticization' thesis in general terms. We need to examine it in more detail here, as it relates specifically to the creation of personhood. It would be all too easy to assume that the progressive identification of more and more conditions with a genetic basis leads inexorably to the redefinition of persons in molecular terms, or the transformation of social relations into genetically defined categories of biological relatedness and shared risk.

Clearly there are indeed tendencies in that direction. The insertion of genetics into a broad array of medical conditions undoubtedly introduces new forms of self-awareness, and the identification of genetic risk has significant implications for individuals who are affected, or potentially affected, and members of their kin. Equally, however, we must be careful not to assume wholesale transformations in this domain. If there is a persistent *longue durée* for the clinic, then there are equally enduring forms of personhood and social relatedness. If medical practice is best thought of as a palimpsest of knowledge-systems and practices, then so too is personhood and so too are social relations.

The idea of biological/biomedical citizenship is a case in point. Promoted by authors such as Rose (2006; Novas and Rose, 2000), this notion has a double valency. On the one hand, it implies that individual and collective identities are increasingly shaped by shared biomedical characteristics. They include shared genetic risk, characteristics defined by ethnicity, shared environmental exposure and an array of features that are simultaneously social and natural. In that sense the contemporary person is rendered increasingly biological. Gender, race, life-span and other life-chances are increasingly identified in terms of biologically given predispositions. So too are character traits, moral character, mental health, even sociability itself. At the same time, however, such biological-cum-medical categories, such as those prescribed by genetic constitution, create the possibility for the emergence of new social formations and new bases for collective action. Biological citizenship may, therefore, imply mobilization in terms of shared interests that are defined in biomedical terms.

We can see a mobilization of lay people around Rett syndrome that displays features of biological citizenship. The processes can be dated quite precisely and the key actors identified. Around the time of the first English-language accounts of Rett syndrome (Rett, 1977; Hagberg *et al.*, 1983) and subsequent papers in the 1980s describing the clinical classification of this syndrome (cf. Budden, 1986; Naidu *et al.*, 1986; Coleman *et al.*, 1988; Kerr and Stephenson, 1986), the first international family association mobilized around this condition. The US-based International Rett Syndrome Association was created in 1984 by 'a determined group of parents' to support families, raise awareness and importantly fund biomedical research, including the team that identified the MECP2 gene in 1999. Following the MECP2 discovery a 'passionate group of parents' broke away to form the Rett Syndrome Research Foundation to focus their efforts on raising money to support a programme of basic biomedical research (their funding programme included Adrian Bird's reversal of symptoms in a mouse model in 2007). The announcement of the rescue experiment had a significant impact on the goals of these organizations and the two groups merged to form the International Rett Syndrome Foundation (IRSF) with a unified mission 'to fund research for treatments and a cure for Rett syndrome while enhancing the overall quality of life for those living with Rett syndrome by providing information, programs, and services'. However, their ultimate goal repeated in all the promotional material is the development of a cure, and typically the chief scientific officer (Horton, 2010) for the IRSF emphasizes this mission within their fundraising campaigns:

> This means a lot of new people will be learning about and hopefully donating to help us conduct research and find treatments to help symptoms and ultimately, reverse Rett syndrome.

The IRSF have harnessed parental social capital to develop their organization. Leading members have expertise in branding, marketing, public affairs, management consultancy, sales, information technology, law and neuroscience, key skills drawn on in the development and operation of this large-scale organization. For example, a typical member of the Board of Trustees is Ed, a professional lobbyist. Following his daughter's diagnosis he worked with (the then) New York Senator Hilary Clinton to increase federal funding for Rett syndrome research. He emphasized his commitment to using his expertise to further that aim:

> Our girls cannot speak for themselves so we must be their voices, working together to fight for recognition and funding to find a cure. Today we must win support to let us provide our daughters the best care possible so they can reach their full potential. That is the mission of IRSF. It fights for our girls by uniting their families. I hope that my legislative and political skills can make the board more effective when dealing with the public sector. Our girls' voices need to be heard in the corridors of power. A strong IRSF will make that possible.

The success of these organizations in funding and directing biomedical research on Rett syndrome can be linked to the early mobilization of parents into the scientific domain. A key personality in this field is Monica Coenraads, who has been at the forefront of driving the scientific agenda towards a cure. Following the diagnosis of her daughter with Rett syndrome she co-founded the Rett Syndrome Research Foundation in 1999 and was their scientific director for eight years. Following the announcement of this key discovery (Adrian Bird's reversal of symptoms in a mouse model), she moved on to co-found the Rett Syndrome Research Trust (2007) as an 'agile, aggressive successor to pursue the next steps from that milestone'.

In addition, there is a large constellation of local and national parent groups (for example, Rett Syndrome Association UK and the Scottish Rett Syndrome Association, and the Italian group, proRETTricercia) and organizations that have formed around this syndrome. They too share the common purpose of raising money to fund basic biomedical and translational research with a goal to find a cure for Rett syndrome.

Social media also allow for the greater involvement of grassroots campaigners working to raise awareness about the syndrome. For example, the Oprah Please

Speak for Silent Angels (OSSA) Campaign run by a 'Mom' who has a child with Rett syndrome. This campaign is organized via a Facebook member page titled with Oprah Winfrey's name to encourage mothers who have daughters with Rett syndrome from around the world to send letters to persuade the programme makers to feature the syndrome in a segment of the show. A few weeks after its launch, over 10,000 letters had been collected. In this context campaigning for a higher media profile is closely linked to fundraising opportunities.

There has been a rapid rise in interactive and user-generated content via Facebook, YouTube and other social networking sites and blogs focused on Rett syndrome. For example Rett.tv gives parents the opportunity to view video clips and upload their own video content of their daughters and their lives, some celebratory, some offering tips and advice, others seeking help and support. The walls of the many social networking pages and sites associated with the syndrome are full of loving celebration of children with Rett syndrome. These are forums where parents share experiences and post messages of support and as in these typical postings, parents also use these sites to make connections with each other:

DAWN: This is our angel, Scarlet. We adore her and her big sister, Evie. Scarlet continues to amaze us every day with her smile and sense of humour. She was diagnosed in August after 18 months with a classic autism diagnosis. We will be going to our first IRSF conference in May. See you there!

SARAH: Dawn, I hope to meet you in May!

CLAUDIA: Scarlet is just precious, thank you for sharing. I look forward to seeing you in May. Have you connected with other families local to you?

There is a plethora of web-based forums with a focus on Rett syndrome. These predominantly contain posts from families seeking support, with others in turn providing advice and reassurance. In response to one mother telling the group about her daughter's hospital admission, another provides support and encouragement: her daughter adjusted to this treatment (a diet for children with difficult to control epilepsy). It is clear that many of these parents contribute to a range of on-line forums and many also have their own on-line presence via personal blogs:

CARLA: Hello! Sienna has been admitted to our local hospital for 3–4 days to start the ketogenic diet. I will be keeping track of our experience on my blog. I posted a link to a recent blog about her seizure history.

DANIELA: We'll be thinking of you. Hang in there. I held my Poppy's hand through this, and she quickly adjusted. Take it one hour at a time.

It would, however, be unwise to assume that this plethora of networks and the visible mobilization of large numbers of parents around this syndrome mean that this had led to wholesale transformations in identity-formation. It is clear that some individuals and alliances can come together on the basis of shared medical interests; however, it is not the case that biomedical categories exert an equal influence on all potential actors. Indeed, as several key sociological and anthropological studies have shown, involvement with genetic conditions does not lead inexorably to a geneticized identity, or to a 'master-status' defined primarily in biomedical terms.

A prime example of this absence of biomedical identity-formation is provided by the work of Bharadwaj (2002; Bharadwaj *et al.*, 2007). This derives from research on a series of informants who had been identified as being genetically predisposed to developing genetic haemochromatosis. Haemochromatosis is a condition characterized by an overload of iron that is stored in the body's organs. If it is identified early, the sequestered iron can be depleted by nothing more sophisticated than regular bleeding. If the condition is not identified – and its symptoms are diffuse – then it can lead to major physical damage and even death. The individuals interviewed by Bharadwaj were identified in the course of routine blood donation. With their consent, blood donors were screened for genetic susceptibility to haemochromatosis. A number of individuals were identified as having the genetic predisposition, and were contacted by the haematology service. A sample were interviewed, together with another sample who had been identified on a clinical basis, and had frank illness. One might hypothesize, on the basis of arguments concerning geneticization and biomedicalization, that the identification of a genetic predisposition on the part of the blood donor group would lead them to experience a sudden threat to or transformation in self-identity. With no reason to assume that there was anything untoward, they went from being morally worthy blood donors to 'risky' people, in the condition of being potential patients.

In effect, the research painted a different picture. Being identified as having a genetic predisposition did not result in such an existential or ontological transformation. On the contrary, many of the respondents adopted a remarkably matter-of-fact attitude. Their expressed attitudes did not provide evidence of a geneticized identity. Nor did the fact that the individuals so identified were being followed up with regular blood-letting appear to result in any transformation on the basis of 'surveillance' or 'governmentality'.

Of course, genetic haemochromatosis does not cover all possible types of genetic conditions, much less can it stand as proxy for all biomedical novelties. On the other hand, it was selected quite deliberately by the social scientists in order to provide a test case for the possible impact of adult population screening for common conditions. And this is one case where a relatively negative (or at least the absence of a florid) finding is informative. Clearly, the evidence shows that genetic risks can impact differently, depending on the condition, its likely severity, the predictability of onset and so on. (Haemochromatosis is relatively unpredictable in its trajectory, unlike some other genetic conditions such as Huntington's disease.) But this is entirely what one would expect, quite apart from arguments concerning biomedicalization.

One cannot assume, therefore, that the identification of a condition as genetic or its biomedical character will automatically give rise to a transformation in personhood or patienthood. While these organizations are formed on the basis of parental mobilization in response to their child's diagnosis, they are run by a small group of highly motivated individuals working towards a cure for the syndrome who also display high levels of social capital. The huge array of online social networks also appeared to indicate the power of a genetic diagnosis to mobilize parents into group activism around this condition. However, many of the parents we spoke to rejected or felt excluded from these networks.

Many parents found their experience of attending conferences and events with a focus on Rett syndrome, and meeting other parents and children, upsetting and something they did not want to repeat. Many did not want to meet other children with the syndrome and to be faced with the future trajectory of their child's condition. For Rebecca, the mother of Phoebe, a six-year-old little girl with a mild version of the syndrome (although she could not speak, she could walk and was very mobile and engaging), attending wider network events and support group meetings associated with the syndrome presented her with a frightening future. It forced her to witness children with a more severe and distressing form of Rett syndrome and some older women with the syndrome. This presented her with an insight into the decisions she would face as her daughter got older such as the provision of long-term care:

> REBECCA: You know, and I'd started to accept who she was and things got better then and I stopped, you know, like sort of – the Rett Association, I stopped that. I stopped all those sort of things because they were frightening me. […] the Rett Association they were so negative, to me it was negative, that I wish I'd never done it because I kept thinking, you know, I kept thinking, for us to sit there, this is what they mean. To have to go into respite care, and I – you know, you're waiting for it to happen.

The family association conferences are promoted as an opportunity for parents to meet and support each other, learn more about the syndrome and the latest research, and to meet the family association team and the clinicians and scientists involved in the syndrome. However, for parents new to the syndrome and with a recently diagnosed child, the conference has another role. Attending the conference also means they experience seeing a large number of children with the condition under one roof for the first time – parents may not have met other children with the same syndrome before. The family conference takes place at a large hotel situated on the edge of a motorway exit. The large atrium is filled with people and there are a couple of tables manned by the association welcoming people, providing conference packs and information and advice leaflets, and also selling books, mugs, tea towels and pens, etc., to raise money, and tea and coffee are served. Within this large hotel reception space people are greeting each other as old friends and it is a communal space where all the children are admired and celebrated. However, there are also a small number of individuals and couples who are set apart, and it is not clear if they are attending the conference or just staying at the hotel. This atrium serves as a space where parents can meet, but it is also a site where parents can place their child more starkly in the spectrum of abilities within the syndrome. While some children are walking and playing and appear to be mildly affected by the condition (although they may not be affected at all, this is a public place and there are families staying at this hotel who are not part of the conference), there are a number of very frail and tiny little girls in buggies who have gastrostomy tubes and clearly have multiple health problems. There are also two older women with the syndrome who are more visibly affected by profound disabilities, one accompanied by carers and the other by much older parents who are in their 70s. These women are wheelchair-bound and have more advanced features of the syndrome, have pronounced scoliosis and have coarser facial features. Parents also come face-to-face with a number of possible futures for their child and for themselves.

Despite these wider family networks and organizations, all the parents we spoke to experienced high levels of social isolation. They were all living and coping with the everyday reality of caring for a child with severe disabilities who needed full-time care and would be dependent on carers for the rest of their lives. It was common for parents to recall that the onset of their child's problems and their subsequent diagnosis led to a narrowing of their social worlds, with many losing friends, and the breakdown of relationships with many divorcing at this time. Jackie describes feeling cast out by her circle of friends who stopped visiting:

> I mean it was so stressful to be – because we really were – cast out. Lots of so-called friends didn't come and visit any more, and I really did, I became quite isolated, and out of choice eventually because I decided that if we weren't socially accepted well damn them, then we're not and we'll do it our way. So we did tend to, the three of us [her and her two children]. I mean my husband was at work during the day, but the three of us tended to just do things together. Fortunately for Jack [unaffected son] he's always been a sociable and a very easy-going child, but one has to say – is he easy-going because he had to be?

Many other families believed they were excluded from these support networks. Some children remain without a name for their condition and are never given a definitive diagnosis because their features are not considered clinically to fit the classic description of the potential syndrome or they have features that lie across a spectrum of syndromes. A failure to receive a definitive diagnosis for their child was also extremely upsetting for many parents. Many described the emotional toll of years of hospital appointments where potential diagnoses were presented and then taken away from their child. For some parents this occurred a number of times, and for many, a definitive diagnosis never materialized. Parents spoke of the importance of seeking a definitive diagnosis, not just for them but also described it as part of their responsibility to their child. Catherine is angry that her daughter (Millie) has not been given a 'definite' diagnosis of Rett syndrome by their clinician. She describes the difficulties of not having a label for her child's problems. Although Millie has many of the features associated with Rett syndrome, her clinical team does not believe it is enough to fit her within the classic pattern of the syndrome. Instead Millie sits at the edges of the syndrome; without a diagnosis she cannot be part of the Rett syndrome community (or any other community linked via a specific syndrome) or access the wider support networks that children with a definitive diagnosis receive. Catherine bitterly describes this as leaving her in 'a bad situation':

> He was reluctant to give a definite diagnosis for Millie. He said at various points, 'She doesn't fit the classic pattern we see.' He said she had Millie's Syndrome in the end. That was his last word. Now, this was a constant barrier to us because I don't know if you're aware but children without a diagnosis are in a bad situation. Yes, if they don't have a diagnosis they fall into this neverland situation and they don't seem to get the amount of support they would if they had a diagnosis.

Catherine goes on to describe the importance of a diagnosis not just for her daughter, but also for her wider family. Not having a definitive name was particularly upsetting for her mother who had been heavily involved in the Rett family associations and raising money for research. However, without her granddaughter having a definitive diagnosis, within these settings she now runs the risk of Millie's diagnosis being queried by other parents and her legitimacy to be part of the Rett syndrome family network being called into question:

> My parents took up the role of going to the review meetings, which we've always done, we've never missed and we've obviously maintained as much contact as we can, and they were doing that for us because we were abroad and my mum found that – I mean her belief was always that Millie had got Rett syndrome, that's why she supported the Association and has done fundraising and that sort of thing, although she obviously thought it was a good cause anyway – and she found it very difficult dealing with people in the meeting who didn't believe that Millie had it.

Without a definitive name for their child's condition parents were not able to claim full membership of patient and family support groups for the syndrome. It meant they were always on the edges of these groups and were always aware that their identity and right to membership might be called into question.

The search for a diagnosis

Parents who did have a child with a definitive clinical diagnosis of Rett syndrome typically described a long drawn out search to obtain a diagnosis or name for their child's problems and all emphasized the emotional toll that this took on them. Many parents expressed a strong need to know and to obtain from their clinical team an explanation or a name for their child's problems. Many parents spent years attending different clinics, seeing a range of clinical specialists and having a large number of assessments and tests carried out on their child and being presented with a spectrum of potential causes prior to obtaining a Rett diagnosis. However, once a name was provided they often found that this did not have any practical positive impact on their everyday life; there is no treatment for this condition and for many families it had powerful negative consequences. Naming their child's problems also defined their child's abilities and the likely future course of their condition and many parents describe this as putting an end to any hopes they had that their child's problems may be treatable or temporary in nature.

Typically, this mother recalls her long drawn out search for a diagnosis that involved visiting a large number of clinical specialists over a number of years (her daughter was 17 years old at the point of diagnosis) to obtain a definitive diagnosis for her daughter. However, she recounts that once she received a definitive name for her child's condition she 'really hit rock bottom'. Although this diagnosis provided certainty – her daughter had Rett syndrome – it also came with the realization that there would be no cure or treatment for her daughter's multiple complex disabilities and that her 'life is not going to change':

> JANE: Once, sort of, we'd fought for her and she was back in school with all her friends again, I think that was when I hit – I just went downhill. And I just sort of was quiet, sitting in the house, crying and wouldn't go out, wouldn't go to town. And in the end I had to admit it that I wouldn't go out. I went to the doctors and was referred for counselling and that made it even worse. Because you're sitting there talking to this person you don't really know and all I was doing, I suppose, was just getting myself all upset. And as I said, my life is not going to change.

The process of receiving a diagnosis often engendered feelings of shock, and this was the case for parents such as Jane above who has spent years searching for a name for her child's condition and for parents such as Nicola below, whose child was diagnosed very quickly once they had become concerned that their child had some development problems. Parents at whatever stage were often still hopeful that their child's problems were temporary:

> NICOLA: Yes, and we've had foster children who've come with huge behavioural problems and emotional problems and hurt, you know, all inside them, not necessarily physically damaged, all those damages, but with time and love and care and everything they could be healed from that. Also I suppose in my mind I believed that any child can be healed if we can help them, and this ... I was being ... I was meeting something that ... No, she's got it forever. I mean you can't be healed from it.

For the majority of parents, diagnosis was not a simple process of being referred to a genetics service and receiving a name for their child's learning disabilities. Some parents received a diagnosis of Rett syndrome for their child's problems relatively quickly once they had been referred to the clinic. But for the majority, the process of attendance at the clinic (or clinics across a range of specialisms) and the search for a diagnosis continued over a number of years. As we have seen, this process did not always result in an unequivocal diagnosis of a specific named syndrome; instead, parents were often provided with a number of potential syndromes that may be the cause of their child's problems or provided with the likely cause and risk of recurrence in future pregnancies.

Thus, there were many hurdles faced by these parents in what was often characterized by them as a long 'battle' with a range of clinicians to receive a diagnosis and name for their child's problems. Almost all the parents we spoke to during interviews, at conferences and at meetings described the search for a diagnosis for their child's problems as lasting many years, punctuated by possibilities, false hope and frustration in their search for the cause of their child's problems, until their child was diagnosed with Rett syndrome. This journey is exemplified by Sue's story of her search for a diagnosis for Jessica. Reading her daughter's extremely large file of medical records at the local hospital, it was easy to see the difficulties they and the medical professionals faced both in caring for Jessica and in identifying the cause of her multiple health and developmental problems.

Sue and Jessica

Sue recalled that everything seemed normal at Jessica's birth and there were no concerns initially about her development. However, at eight months she was admitted by the emergency services into the resuscitation room having had a prolonged febrile fit. Sue recalls:

> When I woke up, I'd got the baby monitor on and she was just breathing funny through it and I rushed into her room and she was just laid there stared up at the ceiling and I don't know how long she'd been like how she was, but she was just a limp rag.

She was seen by a paediatric neurologist and at the time the clinical team noted within the medical records 'some strange breathing and she was pale, jerking her arms and really quite floppy and she continued in that state until she was given some Valium'. Jessica continued to fit, developed pneumonia and was in hospital for a month, during which time the team carried out a large battery of tests including metabolic screening, chromosome analysis, liver function tests, and urine and blood cultures, which were all normal. Following discharge she was readmitted two days later for another two weeks. However, three days following discharge, she was readmitted with a temperature and increased fits and the medical notes record 'rolling eyes, clenched hands, stiff legs, whole body shaking, blueness around lips, jerky, worse on the right side, not woken up properly in between fits, vomited once, not awake enough to take fluids'. A magnetic resonance imaging (MRI) scan showed some atrophic changes in the frontoparietal region of her brain and 'developmental delay' first appeared in her notes. Recalling that time, Sue assumed that these problems were temporary and once the cause was identified they would be resolved or cured:

> Well, we knew something was wrong obviously at that stage, I mean the amount of seizures she was having, we knew she was going to be very behind but we didn't know the extent of the problems but we knew she was always going to be that bit more behind. But at that time I was still thinking, well she's just, you know, she's playing catch-up now, she'll be all right in a few months and ...

However, Jessica's symptoms became progressively worse and at 17 months the medical records note that Jessica was now having episodes of screaming lasting up to three-and-a-half hours and was 'not speaking, not walking, doing lots of eye flicking, not interested in toys but does eat and drink'. At this time, Jessica was having between one and eight fits in a day, all lasting about a minute each, and a typical day was recorded by Sue in her diary at the time:

MONDAY: Seems generally unwell, eyes seem to be flicking a bit more today, mid morning started screaming (1 hour) and then settled down to sleep, slept for 2 hours, which is unusual and then woke up screaming. The pattern of screaming and sleeping continued all day. Didn't eat or drink much, seemed to go red and hot in face, didn't have high temperature. By 8 pm had doctor check her over but didn't find anything, gave Calpol, slept all night, woke up fine in morning.

TUESDAY: Seems very irritable and lethargic, eyes rolling and flicking almost constantly, slept for an hour a.m., when woke, seemed normal for an hour then she started rocking head a lot and eyes started going again. Fingers continued to be in mouth all the time and she has no interest in walking.

During this six-month period Jessica was being looked after by a paediatric neurologist and a wide range of other specialists and had been admitted via the emergency services four times. At this stage Sue became severely depressed, had been prescribed anti-depressants and the medical file records her saying that 'she can't go on like this any more'. During our interview as we discuss this period she becomes visibly upset and finds it hard to talk about this time:

> It was probably that year that I was ... well not ashamed to admit it but I nearly cracked up in hospital. I lost a day; I was in hospital with Lucy and I lost, I don't remember a day. All I remember of that day is my dad coming up and dragging me from the hospital. I don't remember anything else. I remember going down to the car to put a ticket on the car, but I was obviously off the ward for a long time because when I got back everyone was flitting about trying to find me; I'd been gone hours and as far as I was concerned all I'd done was gone down to put a ticket on the car. Where the

> hell I was I don't know [Sue starts sobbing]. Do you know, I've not sat at all until now and thought about that year 'til now and it's just hitting home what I went through. Sorry, I'm all right. It's just hit home [we find tissues and make tea].

She recalls being on her own struggling to cope with her daughter's problems, the large array of medications and regular hospital appointments. She speaks of the strain this placed on her marriage:

> We went through a hell of a rough stage when Jessica was first in hospital because he wouldn't talk to me, he wouldn't tell me what he was feeling. I was going through all that at hospital, I knew what was going on with Jessica as far as the nurses were doing this, that and the other and [paediatric neurologist] wanted this test done and that test done and he, on the other end of the phone, he wasn't part of my life for two or three months or whatever, it just, he just came in of an evening and brought me dinner. He just ... he used to come home, I mean I've found out since then obviously, he used to go to his mum's and sit out on their back doorstep and cry.

Eighteen months after her first hospital admission Rett syndrome and Angelman syndrome first appear in Jessica's medical records as potential diagnoses. However, the paediatric neurologist notes that her hand movements are 'not typical' of Rett syndrome. Jessica is referred to one of the leading (nationally and internationally) centres in child health and this team record that Jessica was 'dysmorphic with coarse facial features and has an unusual head shape'. They agree this is a difficult case and a diagnosis of Rett is a possibility:

> I agree that Jessica does not have the typical features of classic Rett syndrome but suspect that when we have a definitive laboratory test, it will identify the underlying abnormality. Some children who don't have entirely typical features will prove nevertheless to have the underlying biochemical gene abnormality.

They suggest a further referral to the UK expert in Rett syndrome and Jessica receives from this specialist a clinical diagnosis of Rett syndromes at three-and-a-half years old, almost three years after her first hospital admission.

However, for Sue, this is just the first stage of her story. Jessica now had a diagnosis but that confirmed she had profound learning disabilities and would need long-term constant care. Sue is the primary carer for her daughter and has no respite care in place:

> I mean my husband's here, it's not like I'm on my own and ... but he doesn't really have a lot to do with Jessica and her care. She's got a gastrostomy

tube and he won't touch that at all. He won't bathe her. He'll feed her if I ask him to.

Jessica needs round-the-clock care and Sue's daily routine involves getting up on average three times during the night to look after Jessica when she has a fit (during a fit she bangs her head against the side of the bed, which is accompanied by continuous screaming). Jessica also has regular screaming episodes a number of times a week, which can go on for a number of hours at a time. Because Jessica has profound disabilities and cannot communicate or use her hands purposefully, Sue bathes, feeds and dresses her, manages her complex medication (for her epilepsy) and her gastrostomy tube (a feeding tube inserted directly into the stomach) and carries out daily physiotherapy to prevent scoliosis. Spending a day with her it was clear she had time for little else. Since Jessica's problems became apparent four years ago Sue's social life has narrowed, although she has one close friend nearby who also had a daughter with Rett syndrome. She has no respite care because she does not feel comfortable letting anyone else look after Jessica, although occasionally her mother baby-sits for her. When asked to consider the future she was stoical: 'It's my life now, isn't it?'.

Rett angels, locked in by the syndrome

The biomedical discoveries surrounding this syndrome appeared to have had an impact on the ways in which the syndrome was understood and made sense of by parents. The identification of the syndrome as being genetic in origin following the discovery of the MRCP2 gene and the successful reversal of the symptoms of the syndrome in a mouse model appear to have shaped some of the ways in which the family networks and organizations and parents themselves made sense of the ways in which the syndrome affected their child.

As we have seen, fundraising and awareness campaigns typically refer to girls affected with the syndrome as angels and the description of these girls as 'silent angels' is commonly used on a strategic level by family networks and organizations, but also by parents to describe their child. Within the on-line community, parents principally portray children with the syndrome as angels. For example, one site dedicated to awareness-raising has as its subtitle 'dedicated to silent angels everywhere'. Within their posts, parents typically describe their child as 'our Angel' and speak of 'the pleasure of raising a Silent Angel with Rett syndrome':

JENNY: We were blessed with our Rett's Angel seven years ago. Amy can walk and while she can't talk, she signs very well. Our granddaughter is our joy and always brings smiles to anyone who meets her. I hope everyone who is able will support the foundation on the 24th and afterwards too.

The ways in which the syndrome is understood and made sense of by parents and families appear to be closely linked to wider mobilization of images and descriptions of Rett syndrome used by the family associations in their campaigns to raise money for biomedical research. The literature they produce typically represents the syndrome as a condition that traps children within their body. This is particularly visible within their lobbying and fundraising activities targeting government funding for biomedical research; for example, the International Rett Syndrome Association (IRSA) in a press release for one of its annual visits to lobby Congress describe the syndrome as:

> A neurological disorder occurring predominately in girls. It affects girls between ages 6 months to 18 months and renders once happy and playful children unable to communicate and control body movements.

While this does reflect some of the key aspects of the condition such as the period of regression when children with Rett syndrome lose skills such as speech and purposeful hand use, it also suggests more powerfully that this is a type of 'locked-in syndrome', a neurological condition that leaves once-normal children unable to communicate. During one of the international scientific conferences organized by a family association, a parent who is also one of the leading figures in the field ends her introductory address with a clear statement on the focus of the meeting. Her strident tone also gives a clear indication to all present of the acceptable framing of the syndrome within this setting:

> This meeting is dedicated to the girls who live imprisoned in their bodies.

Similarly, publicity material produced by the Italian family association (proRETTricercia) is dominated by appealing and sentimental photographs of children with the syndrome, who we are told are waiting for a cure. In the video a series of beautiful children gaze into the camera and were given a voice describing how the syndrome affected them. The voiceover presents a compelling description, suggesting that this syndrome has trapped this child within her body, unable to communicate. She is waiting for a cure:

> A photograph of a pretty young girl with plaits looking into the camera is given a voice: 'When I was born I was beautiful and healthy, then, after a year, something terrible suddenly happened, but I don't know who did it … the world slipped away from me. I lost speech, I lost use of my hands, but the emotions are still trapped within me. I can't walk, I see the world and I know it, but I can't reach it … '

Prior to onset girls appear to be developing normally but this changes with the onset of the syndrome: they go through a period of regression and lose many of the skills they had, including speech. This allows Rett girls to be described as silent angels, with the syndrome trapping them within their bodies. Thus, the potential of a cure or reversal of the syndrome (promised by the apparent reversal of symptoms of the syndrome in a mouse model) in those affected implies that this could return these girls to the apparently normal state before the onset of the syndrome. This is a potent future promise that has a strong hold over parents.

In our interviews with families, it was common for many to describe feeling that although their child was unable to speak, they were able to understand the world around them in some way. In her account, this mother describes the difficulty of never knowing for certain what her daughter was able to understand or 'take in' about the world. Her account of watching her daughter and looking for any signs of communication and understanding reflects the more general belief among parents that the syndrome traps the girls within their bodies, stopping them from communicating:

> What's fascinating about Daisy is you don't know how much she's taking in. It's really fascinating. It's this – how much does she take in? The video [a simple video game], I mean, on it, you can tell she's comprehending that she's moving it. You just can see the concentration on her face. And she's like – and you can see that she's pressing it and then she'll stop. And it's almost like you'll see the cogs going round.

Many parents described their daughter as locked within her body by the syndrome, waiting for a cure. This supports a hope that one day they will be able to communicate and this mother describes her belief that her daughter is attempting to communicate with her:

> ANNETTE: I'm sure at times she gets frustrated; you can see it when she tries to do something or even just looking at us. She is trying to communicate, look if she is poorly or something like that; for example, she looks at [sister], she looks her in the eye and looks at her dad in the eyes and so it's trying to transmit that 'there's something wrong with me – try and sort something out!' you know.

Without speech, many parents found eye contact the main way in which their children could communicate their needs. Nicola describes how only she can interpret these subtle signs and can read her daughter's communication via smiles and blinks:

> No, I would say the hardest is just that she can't communicate back to you. Because she understands everything, everything you say to her she understands. And she answers by, she either blinks her eyes or she smiles. Or you don't get anything from her at all, you know, she just can be blank sometimes. And it is just hard that she can't say it to you. That's one of the hardest things I find. You know, if she's not very well she can't say she's not very well. And – but, well, the love she gives out. You know, the big smiles and that.

There are broader cultural beliefs in therapies and intensive treatment to improve or cure a wide range of behavioural and learning disabilities in children, from dyslexia through to autism. This pervasive story of parents who struggle against the odds and fight to improve their child's condition is commonly found within parent-led websites that publish parents' stories and promote a range of therapies and educational and behavioural interventions that lie outside biomedical science. While sites such as these often stress that these parent stories are not miraculous and complete recoveries, they predominantly describe parents who have made remarkable progress in treating or curing their severely disabled child – against the odds. These stories have wider impacts on other families with children affected by profound learning disabilities. Elsa describes the struggle of trying to improve her daughter's learning and behavioural problems through an intensive daily regime of therapists and training, which ultimately resulted in no improvement:

> No, but they used to come each week and try to get her to do something, so we used to bring her home from school and then a walker to try and get her to walk. You know, every week you had a task to do with her to say right, if you can get her to do this by next week, it was almost like training a dog. But it was frustrating because she couldn't do it. So you were trying your best to get her to do it and they would say, keep trying. You felt so defeated all the time.

Many parents were not just dealing with the care of their child, but were also trying to manage what they felt were wider cultural and social pressures to be seen to be working towards improving their child's skills, developing their ability to communicate and ultimately finding a cure.

Parental expectations of the potential for improvement in their children can also be seen within the clinical consultations we observed, where families are attending for diagnosis but importantly, also the clinical management of their child. Within consultations, it was not unusual for parents to describe strongly held beliefs in their child's ability to understand and their potential to develop and improve their communication skills. In this consultation, the team attempt to gently modify this mother's expectations that her four-year-old daughter (who has been diagnosed with 'classic Rett's' and is unable to talk, has severe seizures, has little purposeful hand use and has poor mobility) can communicate and can be taught to develop these skills. The mother reports improvement in her child's ability to communicate and is 'optimistic' that she can improve further. She has taken her to a speech and language therapist in the hope that she could learn to communicate through learning a signing system.

GENETICIST: So she's making progress and development?

MUM: A lot of people think I'm optimistic, maybe I'm reading too much into it, but I see certain things that I think, you know, she's definitely come on.

GENETICIST: You can see the potential and are encouraging her to make the most of the abilities she has.

MUM: That's why I asked, like, I went to see our speech and language therapist now and I was saying, like, if we work really hard on signs and things could she learn it? ...

SPR: I think these girls find that quite difficult.

MUM: I didn't mention that, I didn't know. I just asked would she be able to do it. I knew she wouldn't be able to do full signing, and I just wondered if there was something a little more basic than that, just to copy, so that we have ...

GENETICIST: I do think as you say, generally, quite difficult if you've got something that's involving your hands in a very stereotyped way and a very repetitive way that to actually break away from that is quite difficult and quite a challenge.

During this discussion, the physiotherapist sits on the floor playing with the child and encouraging her to grip toys with her hands. She has little purposeful hand use and it appears that the physiotherapist is demonstrating the limits of the child's abilities to the mother during the consultation.

This is delicate emotional work. Within the specialist clinic, one of the key elements in the taking of a case history is asking about the child's ability to communicate. However, if the team considered the parents appeared to have unrealistic or inappropriate expectations, then they spent a considerable proportion of the consultations coaching parents in recognizing the limitations of their child's abilities. Here, a mother tells the team that her daughter can communicate and can make choices:

NEUROLOGIST: And how do you find Abby as a person? Is she quite a happy little girl generally or...

MUM: On balance, yes. Yes, yes. If you give her enough time and present her with two different toys or activities and she will, given enough time, even she does a lot of eye pointing which indicates choice and she's definitely eye pointing.

The paediatrician immediately responds and describes in detail how the syndrome affects the child's understanding, pointing out that even high-functioning girls who have speech, can walk and have good hand use still have 'severe' learning disabilities. She calls on her expertise as the Rett Queen to pronounce that many of the reported cases of girls with Rett syndrome appearing to communicate despite having no speech are fraudulent:

PAEDIATRICIAN: But I think you were talking about things that you have read up in on the Internet and which give the impression of children doing very clever things – I have never seen that. I have seen them on the Internet and have been told and I've had a demonstration at which I was embarrassed because it was clear that people were making this happen.

She stresses the limited communication skills this child has, and encourages the mother to focus on what is 'real' and to work within the limited range Abby can respond to such as contact with people, music and water:

> So, what I try to stress on this subject is that what you want to look for is what the girl will do herself and you can demonstrate how it can be done and you may need to do that quite a lot. But unless she is doing it for herself then it's not real. I think that these young people get most pleasure out of the contact with people and doing things, seeing success from what they have actually wanted to do and I think music is terrific there – working with objects which respond to them. Whether it's water or musical instruments or people who respond and I think that's where the satisfaction comes. Within the sort of very limited communication that Abby has the sensible thought is that her communication is very much based on, 'I want that', 'I'm hot', 'I'm happy'. and dealing with any discomfort or a need. … I guess as you say there's not a great deal there in terms of – of – if you like, deeper thought processes going on.

It was less common for parents to describe their children as having irreversible cognitive damage or being profoundly mentally disabled. Only a few parents we spoke to described their child as having severe levels of cognitive disability. Gabrielle describes her daughter as having a 'low' level of development, and as an 'experiment gone wrong':

> Well, basically, it just means I think that her brain for some reason – Adrian [husband] has explained it to me; he sees it purely as chemicals because he's a chemist – but the chemicals in her brain have never reached the right point to trigger the right responses or development to take her beyond a certain level, which is fairly low. So there's something missing somewhere or some catalytic chemical that needs to be present for something to happen. She's an experiment gone wrong.

Alison describes her daughter's level of cognitive function as similar to that of their pet dog and focuses on caring for her daughter to ensure she is comfortable and pain free:

> It's a bit like trying to imagine what Rocky's [the family pet dog] thinking, you know. You can't do that. I know lots of people anthropomorphize themselves onto animals and Sophie, well, it's almost like what you haven't had you don't miss or whatever. I mean as long as she's kept as reasonably happy in the sense that she's not in pain or anything, well, what more can you do?

Romantic and sentimental images of the child and hope for the future treatment and cure of the condition dominate the wider parent and Rett syndrome community. The aims of the field (to develop treatment and a cure for the syndrome) also have an impact on how parents make sense of the possibilities for their child. For many parents, it was important to keep hope alive; their personal fundraising activities were closely linked to their hopes for treatment and a cure:

JENNY: Be really lovely if they find out how to remove that gene there. Apparently it's just covered over, isn't it, rather than damaged. So I think, well, why can't they uncover it? And if they uncovered it now at this stage in Ava's life [...] would she catch up? But it's really exciting that they're doing so much research. In the summer Ava went for a cycle ride with us and we raised over £1,000. [She talks to Ava who is a tiny frail little girl sitting in a padded bouncer chair.] Do you remember that? You went on Mummy's bicycle? Yes, you went on the seat on the front. We went pedal, pedal, pedal all day, didn't we? Yes, you remember!

The biomedicalization thesis holds that patienthood is changed, and that the classic sick role is superseded, in a movement from patienthood to the social position of the consumer of health care, responsible for health maintenance, and subject to an extended form of medical surveillance. Our own research, and that of others on a series of genetic conditions, suggests once again that this is not an inexorable process. A great many of the individuals and patients we have studied display a classic orientation towards the clinic and towards the embodied authority of the medical practitioner. The parents we spoke to who wanted to receive a name for their child's condition wanted this to come from the clinical establishment. As we have seen in Chapter 3, families sought out clinical expertise, not only to obtain a diagnosis, but also for prognostic information and reassurance about their children and the care they were providing.

Moreover, one cannot assume that biomedical processes, such as diagnostic or predictive genetic testing, will entail wholesale transformations in the relationship of the patient and the clinic. Our own work with individuals and their family members (mainly in South Wales) across a range of genetic conditions leads us to suggest that everyday social life is not necessarily transformed by biomedicalizing processes (Featherstone *et al.*, 2006). Family life is, of course, impacted on by the presence of clinical conditions. Severe developmental delay and problematic development caused by the wide array of genetic conditions known collectively as the clinical field of dysmorphology, for instance, clearly create issues in everyday living, and give rise to a range of social and cultural issues for the parents of affected children. Likewise, genetic conditions create serious problems of everyday functioning, as well as creating issues of family members' moral status (cf. Featherstone, Gregory and Atkinson, 2007). But members of families where there are affected individuals, or members who are themselves carriers or at risk are not automatically 'geneticized' into novel forms of identity and biologically defined personhood. One cannot read off from highly generalized discourse-based accounts to everyday lives. The implications of biomedical innovation for patients, families and others are empirical questions. They are subject to local variation, cultural framing and interpersonal negotiation.

Equally, therefore, one must recognize that the construction and interpretation of clinical entities is not confined to the clinic or the laboratory. Families and domestic settings are themselves sites where everyday phenomena of heath and ill-health, diseases and syndromes, risks and prognoses are generated, shared (or not), interpreted (or not). It is for that reason that we treat 'the family', as a further site for the construction of the syndrome. While biological citizenship as a concept may overstate the case, we recognize that the persistence of the clinic – one of our key themes – implies the persistence of 'the patient'. That is, the persistence of a mode of thought that seeks to interpret the phenomena of medical conditions, within an interpretative framework of mundane reasoning, and that intersects with the clinical perceptions of the clinician in multiple ways.

It is clear, of course, that parents of children with Rett syndrome develop their own interpretations of the condition. We have remarked already on the pervasive imagery of the 'angel' and its connotations. It reflects and reinforces an implicit understanding of the affected child (usually a girl) who is somehow essentially normal, but is locked into a state that is an impediment to her true self-expression and intellectual development (it might, therefore, seem analogous to an otherwise mentally capable person being in a coma). As we have seen, this image has an especially potent effect in mobilizing support for research and clinical applications that might reverse the process and rescue the inner child. There is no biomedical evidence to suggest that this is a likelihood, apart from the rescued mouse we have already described. The biological evidence suggests that there is no cognitive development, and indeed a regression, after a certain age. The child cannot therefore be fully developed 'within' or behind the façade of the syndrome. This idea clearly has a powerful rhetorical function for some actors and activists, however, but it would be wrong to suggest that this is a dominant trope in all parents' understandings of Rett syndrome.

As with sufferers and family members who have first-hand acquaintance with many conditions, lay actors are active in formulating their understandings of Rett syndrome. The sources for those understandings are multiple. As we have seen, activists can become close to biomedical scientists – not least through directly funding the research – and those researchers can present their results to meetings of network members. The latest research and its implications can thus be worked up by the activists themselves and disseminated through the network by means of websites or newsletters as well as face-to-face contact. Equally, interested lay actors are perfectly capable of acquiring textbook knowledge from their reading, from other interested parties, or through their interactions with health professionals. Moreover, these understandings are often refracted through more general lay frames of knowledge. Since Rett syndrome itself is usually a *de novo* mutation, lay actors are not necessarily exercised by the recurrent problems of tracing inheritance patterns, or interpreting carrier or risk values. They do, however, develop their own interpretations of the condition and its causes. In particular, their understandings of development are set within a framework of everyday psychology.

5 Transforming Rett syndrome

The intervention of genetic knowledge to explain Rett syndrome as a genetic condition has wider impacts on this entity. As we have seen, the relationship between genetic science and clinical medicine may not be perfectly aligned, and the identification of the condition is not always straightforward. In addition, there are many interested parties, whose interests may vary and whose expert understandings of the syndrome itself may differ. This transforms the possibilities of Rett syndrome and the ways in which it may be understood. We have seen the mobilization of lay people around Rett syndrome and we now turn to the ways in which parent organizations and biomedical scientists come together to develop a programme of biomedical research in the field of Rett syndrome.

Promoting Rett

The syndrome is simultaneously promoted to policymakers as both a *rare* syndrome and a *common* cause of learning disability in girls. Rett syndrome is listed as a rare disease within the USA Office of Rare Diseases within the National Institutes of Health, even though in other contexts (for example the European Union classification) it is above the threshold needed for orphan designation. It accounts for 2–3 per cent of all severe learning disabilities and is potentially associated with 10 per cent of all profound disability identified in girls and young women, with an overall incidence of about 1 in 10–15,000 girls (Clarke, 1996), making this syndrome a common cause of severe learning disabilities affecting girls. Well timed to coincide with the critical success Julia Roberts had garnered after receiving the Academy Award for Best Actress in 2001 for her portrayal of Erin Brockovich (a campaigning lawyer), the actress went on to testify to congress in a well-publicized lobbying campaign by the International Rett Syndrome Association (IRSA) to ask for increased funding for neurological disorders. This campaign linked the Rett syndrome gene (MECP2) to a wider range of more common disorders 'afflicting millions' ranging from 'autism to schizophrenia'. As the press release from the IRSA described it at the time:

> A small army of parents and friends of patients with Rett Syndrome, including actress Julia Roberts, swept into Washington, DC today to lobby their Representatives and testify before Congress about the need for more research on this debilitating neurological disorder that strikes young girls between the ages of six and eighteen months. The International Rett Syndrome Association (IRSA) is asking Congress for US$15.5 million in funding for research on Rett Syndrome and related disorders.

Promotional and fundraising initiatives align the syndrome to a wider spectrum of neuro-developmental disorders affecting children and young people under the label autism spectrum disorders (ASDs) and pervasive developmental disorders (PDDs). The American Psychiatric Association definition includes autism, atypical autism, Asperger and Rett syndrome, through to conditions mainly affecting young adults and adult populations such as the major mood disorders, suggesting that by supporting the field of Rett syndrome research this may also help to understand these complex disorders. Mutations in the MECP2 gene lead to a deficiency of MeCP2 protein, a protein that is essential for normal brain development. Although the MECP2 gene is primarily associated with Rett syndrome, it may control or modify thousands of other genes and is implicated in many other brain disorders including other genetic syndromes and learning disabilities such as autistic spectrum disorders through to the major mood disorders schizophrenia and bipolar affective disorder.

MECP2 is also an epigenetic mechanism; epigenetics is a growing field that examines the mechanisms that control gene expression. These epigenetic mechanisms can be reset, erased or inherited; and malfunction of these processes has been associated with a range of neurological disorders such as multiple sclerosis and epilepsy, and neurodegenerative disorders including Alzheimer's disease, Parkinson's disease and Huntington's disease. Fundraising campaigns often emphasize that Rett syndrome would act as a 'Rosetta stone' to help 'unlock the mysteries' of many of these other more common and well-recognized conditions:

> Breakthroughs in Rett research will help unlock the mysteries of many other conditions including autism, schizophrenia and mental retardation. We invite anyone with a passion for curing neurological disorders to join our campaign to reverse Rett syndrome.

These wider associations mean that Rett syndrome and the gene associated with it are being studied by biomedical scientists from a range of disciplines, including genetics, neuroscience, biochemistry, molecular and cellular biology, and across a number of clinical specialisms (genetics, neurology, paediatrics, psychiatry). While biomedical scientists working on the syndrome and the gene attend and present their work at their own disciplinary conferences, they also come together at annual international conferences and symposia with a focus on Rett syndrome. These conferences are organized by the leading family associations who raise money to fund much of this programme of basic biomedical science. The majority of delegates are biomedical scientists and clinicians; however, there are usually a small number of parents present including the leading figures in the family associations who hold powerful positions in the field.

Within the scientific conferences speakers often emphasize that studying the syndrome was as a way to understand the mechanisms involved in these other more common neurodevelopmental disorders. The first introductory paper at one scientific conference (given by a recognized clinical expert within the field) presented a history and aetiology of Rett syndrome. In his paper 'Rett syndrome: opportunities for understanding neurodevelopmental disorders' he emphasized that Rett syndrome provided opportunities for understanding other more common disorders, and other speakers in the same panel linked the MECP2 gene to a spectrum of developmental disorders, with one paper posing the question 'Could MECP2 be a major autism gene?'

At these conferences the family associations also present the field with the personal impact of the syndrome to highlight the importance of biomedical research. Their children are displayed to the scientists either by presenting them in the flesh on the conference platform (we have described this in more detail in Chapter 3) or via sentimental photographic images and films screened for the audience. Girls with this syndrome are not particularly dysmorphic or have particularly unusual or distinct facial features. This is unlike many genetic syndromes, such as Down syndrome, for example, which is a well-recognized syndrome causing learning disabilities and has highly visible and distinct facial features. The appeal of young girls with Rett syndrome is an important marketing tool for the field. All the publicity and promotional awareness-raising material throughout the field uses very appealing and pretty pictures of girls with Rett syndrome. A 2007 film made by a European family association is screened to the assembled scientists on the first day of a conference:

> The film starts with a montage of pictures of very pretty young girls smiling into the camera. Soft Spanish guitar music played in the background as the voiceover adds, 'I need your touch, I want to discover life with you, I look at you and open your heart.' A mother talks to the camera: 'Not knowing what you can do for your daughter, I know she's there with her eyes, they know how to express themselves, but I never lose hope because research can help.' A father adds, 'My daughter's eyes really help me, the look in her eyes gives me great joy, she can express things with her eyes. Like a Tamagotchi, she fades away if you don't look after her.' The voiceover concludes: 'By supporting research we have taken an important path for our daughters.'

By giving the 'girls' a voice asking the researchers to help them, the film emphasized the hope parents placed in this scientific field. In response, the biomedical scientists also reflected and promoted this goal in their talks. Typically, at the start of most presentations speakers set out their commitment to relieve suffering and to help these children. A European biomedical scientist starts his presentation examining autonomic function in MECP2-negative mice by giving a personal statement of the impact seeing children with the condition had made on him:

> I haven't got involved in Rett syndrome at all, but having seen these children, the breathing patterns, the agitation. ... I will now.

Speakers place themselves in relation to the syndrome by displaying their contribution to the field. While giving the introductory paper outlining the aetiology of Rett syndrome, a paediatrician emphasizes the recent developments in treatment and their impact on survival rates. He presents his team as playing a key role in the improved quality of life and the survival rates of girls affected by the syndrome:

> Twenty-five years ago Rett was a fatal disorder and degenerative, however, now girls survive into their 40s, 50s and 60s. We are aggressive in our treatment to ensure survival and quality of life

These multiple sentimental images of girls with Rett syndrome emphasized the importance of finding a cure and reflected back to the biomedical scientists a heroic image of their field, working to rescue girls trapped in their bodies unable to communicate with the world. The romantic and emotional stories within these films promoted the importance of translation to the biomedical scientists.

Promoting translation

The theme of translation has assumed a central role in recent biomedical research and scientific policy more broadly and here it also fashions the present and imagined trajectory of this syndrome. Although translation has a number of connotations (Woolf, 2008), the term is used to capture the movement 'from bench to bedside', that is a movement *from* research *to* medical practice. We see here how key groups within the field come together within the scientific conference setting to create and reinforce a trajectory, which frames biomedical research findings in the field as leading inexorably towards a cure for the condition.

An important boost to the field was the rescue experiment, which demonstrated the apparent reversal of the syndrome in a mouse model. This study subsequently became enrolled in all fundraising literature and suggested the tantalizing possibility of a cure on the horizon. For example, this experiment transformed the IRSF's strategy into one of translation and around this time the foundation started to fund translational research, drug discovery and clinical trials. In 2010, they launched a translational research programme (US$4 million) that set out their 'roadmap' to develop therapeutic treatments and eventually to cure and reverse the effects of the syndrome. Announcements of research funding promoted innovation, speed and the translation of research into therapies and funding streams typically became 'inspired' by this study. The urgency of this translational agenda was explicit within the organization's literature and the Chair of the IRSF committee dramatically described the mission of the organization 'to provide care to families, while searching feverishly for a cure of Rett syndrome'.

At the start of the scientific conferences, the agenda was always set out clearly and stridently, with the emphasis placed on collaboration and cure. At one, in 2007, the opening address by the president of a European family association emphasized to the assembled scientists (many of whom received funding from the family networks) that they had an obligation to translate their basic science and deliver a cure. Although the audience were predominantly European, there were also a small number of biomedical scientists from the USA and parents who were leading figures in the international family networks. The president outlined the hard work involved in raising significant funding for biomedical research and emphasized to the assembled audience of scientists that a debt was owed, a therapy was needed 'fast'. Her inspiration for organizing this meeting was the rescue experiment and the leading scientist responsible for this was the star of the show, setting an optimistic vision of a field working towards a cure:

> We need to collaborate, they need a therapy and need it fast – they need a therapy! We took on the important task of putting together a group who want to find a solution and find it fast. Let me introduce Adrian Bird, his agreement to come one year ago, it spurred us on to organize and run this conference!

She set out the importance of collaboration but also emphasized the division of labour: while families coped with the syndrome at home by looking after their daughters, the scientists must work for the girls in the laboratory:

> It's good to join forces, Adrian Bird's work on disease reversibility will give great impetus to find a new solution leading hopefully to a treatment. We need a strong directive, this is what we ask you, we are aware that a lot of money is needed, that's why we are here, we want to see if there was an opportunity and ask you for more though, you are taking the decisions in the lab, we are tackling it in the home – it is very hard to adapt, it's very painful. And we know it's very hard for you to understand, we are indispensable and important for the life of our little girls.

This speech was a clear moral directive to the assembled scientists reminding them that it was their duty to use the money raised by the family associations wisely and to build on this breakthrough to deliver a cure. The rescue experiment introduced a renewed urgency into the field and legitimated working towards translation. The biomedical scientists also reinforced this story of Rett syndrome and reflected back to parents their commitment to collaboration and translation. Developments within medicine often imply a process of translation and within the conference circuit the field was consistently presented by speakers as one in which the current phase of basic blue skies research would lead the field towards a biomedically driven cure. A powerful rehearsal of this insider story was given by one of the leading biomedical scientists in the field. His presentation reflected this story, focusing on the hope that his research findings (he had just published the reversal of Rett syndrome in a mouse model) would 'reach up towards' the development of a treatment to reverse the syndrome in girls. He further aligned his position with that of the family associations, and described being 'profoundly affected' personally by the possibilities of translating his work into the clinic:

> I too have been profoundly affected – with the hope that my blue skies work can become clinically relevant. I start at the molecular level and try to reach up towards the medical level, it started as a purely basic interest in this mutation in this DNA.

He was clearly enjoying the power his research findings had over the audience, the room was full and everyone was eager to hear more details. He described the results of the experiment as a 'surprise' and focused on the difficulties of making the experiment work; many of the mice used in the experiment died and achieving the right levels of MECP2 expression was extremely difficult to calibrate. He focused his presentation on the mice used, how they were built and how they developed a scoring system to rate the expression of symptoms associated with the syndrome before and after the experiment to demonstrate that 'function is rescued':

> You want to hear about the reversible experiments that were a surprise to you and were also a surprise to us!! We build mice without MECP2 and put it back. We changed the gene to stop the expression, you never know with living things until you do it. [He explains how they carried out the experiment.] Half die and half are cured, it's a kill or cure remedy. Too much MECP2 may be as bad as too little, the over expression of the gene is bad, the cells can't cope in the same way and it leads to death […] We developed a scoring system for MECP2 mice. Before treatment they [mice] were starting to get bad symptoms, tremors, breathing arrhythmia. Afterwards the same animals were remarkably changed, you get pretty good reversal. As you can see on the movie [the video showing the reversal experiment], function is rescued.

He introduced the strategy of translation and emphasized that this finding had 'therapeutic implications' and may translate to reverse the effects of the syndrome in affected girls. Suggesting that although Rett causes neurons to be 'crippled', they do not die, presenting the possibility of reversal:

> The results have obvious therapeutic implications for Rett syndrome. Rett syndrome is not strictly a neurodevelopmental disorder or neurodegenerative.

> Data suggests that they are deficient in maintenance and stability problems of neuronal function. So, if MECP2 is restored, do symptoms disappear? In neurodegenerative conditions neurons die and if they die you need to replace them. BUT there is no sign of neuronal death in Rett syndrome.

After seeing the video of the rescue experiment, questions from the audience focused on translation. The scientist appeared reluctant to give a definitive answer, giving the time frame for achieving translation as anywhere from five to 50 years away. However, he emphasized that he was working towards being the first in the field to achieve this: 'We are busting a gut to be the first!' This is an extremely useful device for biomedical scientists in the field; it validates their call for large amounts of money to carry out basic biomedical research in the field, but also provides a clear justification for continued large-scale funding. Half way through the conference, he uses his position as Chair of the session to emphasize the importance of continued funding for basic biomedical research:

> The field is romping along but it has a way of romping before any treatments. There is still an enormous amount of developments in the field to be made […] it requires the importance of research that doesn't necessarily directly relate to Rett. There is still a role for basic research, it doesn't have to be with patients to make a contribution to the field.

Later that day this became the key topic of discussion amongst conference delegates over drinks in the grounds of the hotel. A group of senior biomedical scientists discussed the rescue experiment with excitement: 'Before we never dared … hoped to look, now we can!' This finding was a profound event for the field and provided these biomedical scientists with a strategic opportunity to promote and repackage their work in the context of translation. It enabled them to justify looking to the future and to claim their work had the potential to be translated into a treatment and possibly a cure.

Tensions in the field

However, this alignment is not without its tensions. As we have seen, while speakers from the family associations are extremely forceful in their promotion of translation and demands for a cure in their presentations, the majority of biomedical scientists took a more cautious approach, emphasizing the role of basic biomedical research. Backstage there was less confidence that this trajectory was realistic. A senior US biomedical scientist was clearly unhappy with the claims made about the rescue experiment and the promise of a cure. She talked quietly and said what had not been expressed in public at the conferences: the key rescue experiment had not been replicated and although the 'big names' within the field were successfully publishing, she did not believe this justified the trajectory of progress and the claims of a potential cure within the field:

> It's [the rescue experiment] a great experiment, but ... they published the one big paper in *Science* but no one can replicate it! [...] The big names are publishing, but they are not all that!

When speakers exceeded the boundaries of what was deemed acceptable by the scientific audience, we glimpsed some of the tensions for the field in maintaining a cohesive story and the ways in which this is policed. A presentation by a biomedical scientist relatively new to the field examined the relationship between BDNF (brain-derived neurotrophic factor is a protein that helps the survival of neurons and encourages the growth and differentiation of new neurons and synapses) and MECP2 in a mouse model. After describing his research findings he stridently emphasized the potential to use this as the basis for a therapy to treat girls with the syndrome. His presentation was consistent with the story of translation, presented earlier at this conference, and he stressed that the increased understanding of the syndrome provided hope for translation into 'new therapeutic targets'. Hope was repeatedly emphasized within this very positive presentation; however, the actual therapies that might be developed remained vague and the timeframe, although 'hopefully soon', was countered by the uncertainty of the field; he of course could not say when this translation into therapies might happen:

> Does this give us hope for new therapeutic targets? I think surprisingly, yes! We now have some tools ... We are actually very hopeful that this type of basic research will in fact lead to the identification of new therapies for the girls, hopefully soon, but we don't know when.

For individual biomedical scientists, aligning their research explicitly within this story of translation can have advantages and this strategy appeared to have fast tracked this speaker to the inner circle of power and funding. During this conference it was noteworthy that he was often seen deep in conversation with a powerful figure in one of the leading family associations funding basic science. However, the scientific audience was clearly hostile to this new insider and delegates aggressively questioned him with a large number of detailed and technical questions – it was clear the audience believed he had gone too far. Although he appeared to be out of step with his biomedical colleagues, his story was extremely attractive to the family networks and appeared to increase his chances of obtaining funding. Delegates such as this US senior biomedical scientist were aware of the fundamental tensions of their alliance with family networks that control funding streams and expect a cure to be delivered:

> Families want a cure so they keep funding the top names, but they are just interested in self-promotion, they should support more junior posts – they

are the future. … It's great working with family associations, it gives you great access to patients, but families control the money so that leads to a focus on a cure.

There appeared to be close links between the leading members of the family associations and the senior biomedical scientists in the field. These relationships and collaborations were visibly displayed to the audiences at these conferences both formally and informally. The leading biomedical scientists were enrolled in the organizing committees of the meetings, their work was presented and celebrated strategically; for example, during the final conference address it was usual for them to be singled out and presented with gifts and awards. They were also predominantly seen in the company of the leading figures in the family associations at coffee breaks and sitting at the 'top table' at conference dinners.

The family associations raising money to fund biomedical research were keen to position their organizations as a resource for biomedical scientists and to bridge the scientific and parent communities, describing their organization as a tool for collaboration, a 'clearing house, helping you to share so that you don't have to reinvent the wheel' and a way for biomedical scientists to share resources and information. The influential head of one family association presented an unproblematic vision of collaboration where biomedical scientists share resources and information, and work together towards a common goal:

The idea is making lists for researchers trying to share reagents, discussing technical problems and even more importantly to collaborate and develop networks for grant applications to keep in touch and to share information.

However, backstage some delegates at a 2005 conference greeted the presentation of the field as a collaborative endeavour with scepticism. Some expressed their reluctance to collaborate; working together appeared to come at a price. While one of the key mouse models in the field was freely available for other biomedical scientists working on Rett syndrome, some complained that the other key model was not available freely, and to use it research ideas and publications had to be shared with the owner. Others spoke of papers being held back from publication by reviewers who were also rivals and a US assistant professor described the field as a closed shop where a small number of people controlled the field:

It's a closed shop, you have to work with one or the other [the two lead scientists at the meeting] and then you get published, I worked in [a childhood genetic condition] before, it was just the same, I'm not in the inner sanctum.

The rescue experiment represents an important moment in the field. It is used to support and shore up the idea that the basic biomedical research within the field has the potential to be translated into a therapy, explicitly framed in terms of a cure. It also legitimates the continued funding of the field, with an emphasis placed on basic biomedical research to drive and push this agenda forward. However, we can also see the tensions this framework produces for the field and for individual scientists.

Creating Rett for research

Calibrating and measuring Rett syndrome for the purposes of biomedical research is another significant site where the syndrome is fashioned. In the scientific conference a range of devices were used to see and manipulate the syndrome: in the bodies of patients observed variously in the flesh, via video and photographic representation and through animal models where the syndrome is also produced, manipulated and reduced. As we have seen, at the start of scientific meetings it was usual for live cases, the 'girl with Rett syndrome', to be presented to the assembled audience to demonstrate the clinical presentation of the syndrome; this also placed the effects of the syndrome on the child and the family firmly in the spotlight. This was also achieved variously via sentimental photographic images and video celebrating the child, presented by the family associations. Within presentations images of children were used in order to classify features and to see the syndrome. However, the majority of the presentations focused not on the child but on the syndrome, using animal models to visualize and manipulate the gene.

Creating a model of Rett for experimentation

Mice are considered the 'gold standard' animal model in biomedical science and are the most common vertebrate species used to build disease models and to map and isolate genes as a short-cut to identify corresponding genes and their function in humans. Knock-out, knock-in or transgenic (DNA from another organism) mice have specific genes inserted, modified or removed in order to mimic or represent a disease, a disease pathway or the underlying molecular mechanisms. A range of Rett syndrome mouse models have been built without functional MECP2 (Chen *et al.*, 2001; Guy *et al.*, 2001; Shahbazian *et al.*, 2002; Pelka *et al.*, 2006). The male MECP2-deficient mice typically have a stunted body and small brain, develop tremors, hind limb clasping, irregular breathing, and usually die within 6–12 weeks following birth (Chen *et al.*, 2001; Guy *et al.*, 2001). The demonstration of the mouse model was key to many scientific papers delivered at these conferences.

The majority of speakers used slides and video to show built knock-out mice within the laboratory, for example in a cage, or performing an experiment such as a maze or memory test; or sections of mice would be presented on slides displaying cross-sections of brain or tissue. However, speakers also found other ways to represent the mouse. One speaker presented the knock-out mice he had used as cartoons, wearing white coats and working as scientists in a laboratory, while the wild-type control mice were represented wearing large sombreros and gun holsters to look like bandits loose in the countryside.

The representativeness of the mouse models used within the field were never called into question at these conferences and it was common for speakers to seamlessly switch between the description of their mouse models and the child with Rett syndrome in their presentations. Throughout her presentation, a Japanese clinical expert described by a delegate at this 2005 conference as 'the Japanese Rett Queen' switched fluidly between the animal and child. She repeatedly emphasized that the knock-out mice she used had clinical and behavioural features of the syndrome that were 'similar to the girls', the mouse 'replicates' the syndrome: 'We are looking at the hippocampus and neuron developments in the brain of MECP2-null mice.' She described the clinical features of the mice without MECP2 as displaying key clinical features to girls with the syndrome:

> These mice are similar to the girls, at 3–5 weeks they are pre-symptomatic, at 6–9 weeks they are symptomatic, clasping, ataxia, seizure-like behaviour. So the MECP2 mouse behaviourally replicates the delayed onset and symptoms observed in human patients.'

A particularly strident version of this was given by one of the leading scientists in the field who had created one of the first and most widely used mouse models. During her paper at the same conference, she stridently pronounced that the phenotypic presentation within her mouse model and the human 'are the same'. To demonstrate this point she played a video of a tiny mouse in a cage; its whole body was shaking severely and uncontrollably. She described this mouse as displaying some of the key features of Rett syndrome in a child; the 'paw clasping' represented hand stereotypies and the uncontrollable shaking a sign of epilepsy in this mouse:

> The mouse and human phenotypes are the same, they are normal at 2–3 months, then they display forepaw clasping and bite when handled, and they can be more severe and have seizures.

However, what constitutes the key clinical features of Rett syndrome appears to be modified in this context. While hand stereotypies are a central clinical feature of the syndrome, breathing irregularities, epilepsy or EEG abnormalities are supportive features and are not central to a diagnosis of classic Rett syndrome (Rett Syndrome Working Group, 1988). However, in the context of the mouse model the pronounced physical features it displayed *become* the syndrome. The mouse paw clasping and the uncontrollable shaking reveal the inner molecular change and become the key physical signs of the syndrome:

> Why Rett's? Well we have mice, it has symptoms which can be expressed in the mouse, e.g. seizures, abnormal gait, breathing. So not only at a cellular level in the brain but also physically – seizures, altered gait – it's got the phenotype as well.

The validity of the Rett mouse models used also depends on the stability of the disease entity itself. Which features need to be replicated, in what combination, depends on how the disease is described, how it is classified and what features are treated as core features. It is not just the mouse that is the model, but also the disease category itself that is being shaped. These models become a further version of Rett syndrome.

Calibrating Rett for research

The work of the local scientific team was a significant site where we could observe the everyday practicalities in the production of an operational and stable model of Rett syndrome to use in their research programme. Within this setting Rett syndrome became increasingly less stable and resistant to classification in the context of their research goals.

The team hoped to increase the identification of cases of the syndrome by improving the associations between the genetic test results (the genotype) and the clinical classification of the syndrome (the phenotype) and to identify new mutations that could be associated with the syndrome. They were searching for new mutations in girls with classic Rett syndrome, particularly in the 25 per cent of cases classified clinically in which no mutation had been identified, and atypical cases where a MECP2 mutation had been identified. They were also looking for rare familial cases by examining families where there was a child with a MECP2 mutation who had a relative with a potentially related phenotype, such as an intellectual impairment, neurological disability or a psychiatric disorder. They hoped this work would eventually lead to the development of guidelines for clinicians on the appropriate use of MECP2 mutation testing. The team had just taken over a national Rett syndrome database classifying a cohort of patients with a clinical diagnosis of Rett syndrome, which they planned to develop by identifying new cases via clinicians who referred cases to their specialist clinic and diagnostic laboratory, as well as through research collaborations.

To develop their expertise in the syndrome and to increase their scientific capital, the team needed a collection of a well-classified cohort of types and cases of this syndrome. The foundation of their research programme was this database (which had been set up by the UK expert in the syndrome) in order to carry out a detailed analysis of the relationship between specific mutations and the clinical features. However, once they obtained and started to examine the database the team found that it was not usable in the ways they had imagined. The classification of the syndrome had changed over time and some key features of the syndrome had not been collected within the original parameters of the database questionnaire, leaving significant gaps in the data. As they continued to discuss this, the team all appeared increasingly frustrated and the senior biomedical scientist emphasized the importance of ensuring they had a robust data set:

> We need to check the spread and look at the gaps, the data is not complete … the value will depend on its completeness.

The collection of cases had a wider function for the team in terms of increasing their expertise and status; having well-characterized data on a large number of cases can enhance their scientific and clinical capital, ensure they become known as experts in the field and become the basis for future research and collaborations. They planned to expand the database by developing their own criteria of features to record and discuss the key diagnostic criteria they need to incorporate in collecting and classifying cases in order to create a robust database. The team had an initial list of items collected by the UK expert who had given them the database: birth and current head circumference, age of regression, abnormalities at birth, congenital disorder, continuing preserved speech, speech level before regression, walking, never walked, hand skills, epilepsy, height. The original database was designed to rank patients' physical ability by combining their score on a number of features: walking ability (5 no limitation to 1 wheelchair use), sitting ability (3 sitting independently to 1 cannot) and hand use (8 ability to pick up objects to 1 no hand function) as a proxy measure for severity.

However, if the team ran into some problems, how could they classify and standardize their description of the clinical features of the sample so that they could carry out an analysis that provided a robust representation of the syndrome? How should they make sense of the variability in the expression of features in children where there is a wide range of phenotypic expression both between children with the syndrome and also within individuals over time? For the purposes of the database (and future statistical analysis) these features needed to be expressed numerically and they faced the challenge of how to reduce complex clinical and behavioural features and transform them into data that could be statistically manipulated. The team spent an afternoon discussing this and clearly became frustrated as they tried to find a more 'objective' way of classifying the syndrome for the database. The discussion continued: 'How do we score to map the diagnostic criteria to capture the variance *and* ensure it maps onto the genotype?' The team considered closely the original scoring system used to rate the clinical features of each child in the database. This used a Likert scale for scoring severity: General mood (1–16), Breathing problems (0–10), Hand behaviours (0–12), Repetitive face movements (0–8), Body rocking (0–14), Night-time behaviours (0–6), Fear/anxiety (0–8), Walking/standing (0–4), etc. They discussed the limitations of these measures and also started to consider their accuracy in representing this entity. What did some of these categories such as 'night-time behaviours' mean in the context of the syndrome where this is not a central part of the classification, and how could they objectively rank behavioural features such as 'fear' and 'anxiety'? The senior clinician added:

> I don't feel this gives us anything useful, these are crude measures, we shouldn't be enslaved by it.

SPR: But we can't be sure of this, we need to make what we can of this data clinically. Can we be more objective?

> [They all look closely at the lists of clinical features in their printouts and are silent for a few minutes.]
>
> SENIOR CLINICIAN: This may not be accurate either!
>
> [Laboratory scientist sighs loudly.]

In addition, medical conditions and their signs and symptoms are not static; Rett syndrome is also characterized by a number of clinical stages and a range of clinical features that change over time in each child. The team discussed how they might account for age in their analysis, particularly when many of the younger children within their sample had been classified but did not yet display key features of the syndrome that develop in older children (for example, scoliosis):

> The team discusses a pressing issue with the database, how do they account for age in their analysis, particularly given that 'the full clinical picture may not emerge until 10 [years old] or even later'? The lead suggests they 'either check each variable for age association [and if they find an association] we should control for them as far as possible in the analysis' or they could 'examine the genotype/phenotype in a sub-sample'.

Many of the central features of the syndrome that are classified within the database are based on subjective measures and the team had to rely on data provided by other, often non-expert sources such as parents or clinicians who may not have any expertise in the diagnosis and recognition of the syndrome. Some of the key features collected within the database are contested within the field and the team considered how to treat the classification of children with the label 'epilepsy'. As we saw in Chapter 3, the team had recently been coached by an expert in Rett syndrome to be far more cautious before labelling a child with a diagnosis of epilepsy. However, the database not only classified epilepsy within the sample, but used it as a key variable in the assessment of 'severity' within the sample:

> [The team carries out a factor analysis in an attempt to identify sets of features within the sample that can be used to account for 'severity'. They go through all the factors that emerge; however, epilepsy is the key significant factor that emerges in the analysis.]
>
> SPR: Epilepsy could be driving these things?
>
> LEAD BIOMEDICAL SCIENTIST: I'm not sure about these diagnoses, it sounds like about a quarter of these vacant spells are being over treated.

The challenge of transforming not just the syndrome, but also the features of each child within their database creates many problems for the team. To represent the case and the syndrome they must read the complexity of the features but also reduce them.

Aligning the clinical and molecular findings

The team also collected photographs and video of the children they were adding to this database in the hope that they would be able to improve the alignment of the inner with the external features and manifestations of the syndrome in the body and face of the child. They believed they would be able to connect the specific mutation in the MECP2 gene to the level of severity and align them to specific physical and behavioural features in the child. Rett syndrome is not associated with a strong dysmorphic facial 'look', but it does have distinct behavioural features: repetitive hand movements that typically develop following the period of regression and autonomic breathing. However, the team hoped that by collecting and classifying a large cohort of patients they would be able to identify a 'face for Rett'.

The SpR had assembled a large set of photographs of children diagnosed with Rett syndrome (or suspected Rett syndrome) as part of her role working up and collecting cases for the database. She was keen to find a look for the syndrome and organized a meeting with experts in the diagnosis and recognition of genetic syndromes that are associated with learning disabilities. The group included two senior dysmorphologists and four juniors who had been working with the consultants as part of their training to become specialists in clinical genetics. The SpR was sitting at the front of the seminar room with a slide projector and screen and introduced the session:

> Thank you all for coming, and being so helpful. What we're going to try and do today is to look at dysmorphology in Rett, and to see whether there's a face for the Rett child, even if they're not dysmorphic and what if it, if there is a face, what makes a face?

She had divided her collection of photographs into three sections by age groups, by mutation type (a number of mutations have been identified) and into a mixed group where the audience had to guess if the child had a diagnosis of Rett or some other syndrome. She quickly flicked though all the slides, which were presented in batches of five to six photographs of faces on each slide. Within each section the photographs were also grouped by age from birth to 7 months, 1–3 years, 4–7 years, 8–12 years, 16–20 years, and then 20 upwards. She asked for no conferring within the group and asked them to write down their thoughts on assessment sheets she had provided:

> Yeah. Are they, are they, do they have consistent features as a group, or not? And if you do see any of the pictures in the groups as ages …

The first selection of slides grouped the children by age and the audience all commented on the variable quality of the photographs. While many were obviously taken in the clinic or during home visits by the team, some had been provided by parents from their collection of family photographs, so some were of christening or birthday celebrations which did not make it easy to see the facial features of the child in detail. The group's overriding response was that they could see no consistent feature or 'face' in this group, and one of the consultants sighed, 'There's such a mixture, isn't there?' The group focused mainly on the significance of eyes and eyebrows, and the overlap with another syndrome, Angelman syndrome. One commented on the shape of the mouth (prominent philtrum, which is the central depression between the nose and the upper lip, and extremely flat thin lips), but added that she could not find a consistent feature, while the most senior member pronounced that she could see a number of features within the sample that were dysmorphic; however, she was also clearly frustrated that these features were not consistent across the sample:

> I felt a lot of them had deep-set eyes, or very long eyebrows, very prominent philtral pillars. So there were a few things that I thought were, sort of, consistent, sometimes you, you know …

As we saw with the other physical and behavioural features of the syndrome, another confounding factor was that children's features change over time. Features associated with the syndrome that were prominent at a young age can disappear or may only develop as the child gets older:

> The other thing is that they change as they get older, and I've found that, I mean, a lot of them have a – I mean, again, not all of them. Some of them had, like what I would call a pointy chin … And when you get older, it vanishes. [They all speak at once, all clearly frustrated.]

The majority did not appear to have particularly dysmorphic or abnormal features and looked 'pretty normal'. The focus on scrutinizing photographs highlighted to the group the importance of the behavioural features associated with the syndrome (hand stereotypies and autonomic breathing), which they felt they might more easily pick up 'if I saw them in the clinic'. They all agreed that although they could identify a number of features associated with an underlying genetic syndrome within the sample, they found many of the girls to be particularly pretty and attractive:

> And that one over the top left looks entirely normal.
> Later on she's a very striking and pretty little girl.
> Yeah, yeah.
> She was, I remember her.
> And the eyes together. She's also very, you know, pretty and normal you know.

However, they all agreed that despite the difficulty in identifying any specific feature or facial 'look' with this syndrome, 'there is something there'. They held an expectation that they would be able to see a face for this syndrome, if not now then in the future when they had seen more cases:

> So, were you feeling funny that the eyes, with the eyebrows, if you used them together, then maybe you can see something?

We have explored just some of the difficulties faced by the local team to develop a stable model of Rett syndrome and their attempts to classify and align cases with biomedical markers. The classic textbook description of the syndrome is a simplified one as was their original non-specialist hopes of achieving their research goals. The more the team learned about the syndrome, the less certain became the clinical description. Their increasingly specialized knowledge meant they had to manage much greater variation and instability within the syndrome and the population of cases, which they found hard to resolve.

Conclusion

The identification of a mutation associated with Rett syndrome allows us to examine the ways in which genetic discoveries can lead to renewed interest by biomedicine in uncommon diseases and syndromes. We have seen some of the ways in which the interests of different fields of biomedicine have focused variously on the gene, the mutation, the protein or the epigenetic mechanism and align around the syndrome.

We have described here the ways in which the syndrome is subject to a close and detailed observation by biomedical scientists in order to read and interpret significance. The visual culture is significant; the syndrome must be seen in the child but also in the models. Sentimental images of the syndrome persist within the sphere of fundraising, but also at the conference itself. In this setting the theme of translation and the goal of rescuing girls trapped in their bodies unable to communicate with the world is both presented and reinforced by the scientific field and parent organizations.

However, the alignment of family groups raising money for research and biomedical scientists is not without its tensions. While in public this trajectory of translation and cure was presented as an achievable goal, backstage there was less confidence. As we have seen, while speakers from the family associations are extremely forceful in their promotion of translation and demands for a cure, the majority of biomedical scientists take a more cautious approach.

Importantly, the syndrome must be calibrated to produce a standardized version for the field. However, attempts to standardize the disease and the patient have proven extremely difficult – the more the local team examined their sample, the more they found a wider range of variability and instability provided by the local practices in naming, classifying and interpreting. The identification of a genetic basis does not remove all ambiguity concerning the classification and description of Rett.

6 The making and remaking of medical classifications

We conclude this work by picking up, recapitulating and developing some of our key analytic themes. Rett syndrome has intrinsic interest, and its significance for affected children and their families cannot be exaggerated. But our own analytic perspectives are intended to go beyond this one, relatively uncommon, condition itself. We have chosen to document some of the social processes and events surrounding it because it illustrates some more pervasive aspects of contemporary medicine, and of key sociological or anthropological perspectives on it.

In general terms we have emphasized, and illustrated, a number of recurrent themes. Throughout this monograph we have repeatedly stressed the multiplicity of Rett syndrome itself. Notwithstanding its undeniable medical and biological basis, the condition does not exist *as* 'Rett syndrome' independently of the work of identification and interpretation that go into its production and reproduction. That work is enacted in multiple sites and settings, and we have followed the condition through them. We have emphasized that the syndrome is neither fixed nor a single entity. It changes over time, and it is constructed in different versions. Those range from the journal science of contemporary biomedical research, to the performance of clinical judgment, the work of activist coalitions or the everyday interpretations of parents and family members.

Rett syndrome has a particular significance, because it is one of the many conditions that have been identified as having a genetic basis. It thus exemplifies some processes that are identifiable across a wide range of conditions and medical specialties. It is one of the many clinical conditions that are implicated in the rise of the new genetics, and the growing significance of genetic medicine within the wider domain of biomedical knowledge. Our multi-sited ethnography of Rett syndrome is, therefore, intended to be a contribution to the much wider scrutiny of genetic medicine and its scientific and cultural significance.

Our focus is on medical conditions that are currently identified in genetic terms, which reflects our particular interest in medical genetics. However, we do not intend to convey the impression that these processes are unique to genetic conditions. We do not privilege genetics in this context. Equally, our focus on genetic conditions has a point: that an ever-increasing number of conditions are being defined as having a genetic cause or a genetic component is one important, contemporary example of how medical conditions are available for successive phases of definition and classification. The current state of genetic medicine is not an end-point in these processes of construction. It is a distinctive phase in a historical and cultural process, and it has some distinctive characteristics. It is not, however, the culmination of an evolutionary process, nor the end-point of a progressive revelation of biomedical truth. Indeed, our argument has some urgency precisely because of the need to resist any implication that genetically based biomedical explanations mark the *end* of classificatory redefinitions. Indeed, it will be one of our themes here to suggest that recent interventions based on medical genetics have often destabilized medical definitions.

Rett syndrome displays many characteristic features of the trajectory of a genetic condition (cf. Brown, 1995). The original identification and naming of the syndrome reflects a common pattern. It was, as we have said, first identified from a small series of cases by one clinician. Rett originally referred to it as 'puppet syndrome', reflecting the characteristic appearance and behavioural characteristics of the children. The attribution of descriptive or exotic names to such syndromes has been common: examples from the general field of dysmorphology and developmental delay include cri du chat syndrome (based on children's characteristic vocalization) and Kabuki syndrome, so called because the facial features of the individuals resemble the make-up of Japanese Kabuki actors. These features include long palpebral fissures of the eyes (a narrowing of the space between the upper and lower eyelids), arched 'interrupted' eyebrows and prominent eyelashes, giving the impression that the patient is wearing eyeliner. The subsequent adoption of the label Rett syndrome of course also reflects the common adoption of an eponymous clinician who first identifies the condition. At this point in its trajectory, the syndrome is defined primarily in clinical terms – that is, by reference to the characteristic signs of developmental delay, the child's physical appearance, and the typical repetitive hand movements. Symptoms such as disturbed breathing patterns or epileptic-like episodes may be associated clinically with the condition, but are not treated as a defining (pathognomic) feature.

Without a name, and the description of a type-case, no distinctive clinical entity can conceptually emerge from the plethora of possible symptoms, explanations and appearances. On the other hand, the act of naming a condition can, of itself, imply a distinctive claim. It not only lays claim to the distinctive existence of a given condition (sometimes a big claim in itself), but also stakes a claim in what *manner* of condition it might be. The original description of the syndrome and its subsequent representation in 'textbook' medicine located it among the other conditions of problematic physical and cognitive development. In terms of a medical specialty, it fell firmly within the province of 'dysmorphology', a specialist field of practice that encompasses a very large number of syndromes and diseases, many of which are rare, but which give rise to a florid collection of types. Over 3,000 conditions and syndromes have been described (London Dysmorphology Database [LDDB], 2000; Pictures of Standard Syndromes and Undiagnosed Malformations [POSSUM]; Jones, 1997).

The key turning-point in the short trajectory of Rett syndrome (it being of recent origin) resides in its identification as a genetic condition. As we have seen, the identification of MECP2 as the site of the genetic anomaly responsible for Rett transforms the condition into a new kind of entity. This is, in other words, not merely the addition of a new cause or origin for the syndrome, it is a transformation in the kind of condition it is held to be. It also invests the syndrome with a new significance, and renders it relevant to new biological and medical specialists – in medical genetics. It also, of course, introduces new modes of diagnostic investigation. It makes it possible for the medical team to undertake molecular tests in order to identify or eliminate the presence of the MECP2 mutation in a patient.

Two related things might be taken to follow. First, it is tempting to extrapolate from this key event that Rett syndrome has become purely 'geneticized', and therefore subsumed under the novel discourse of *biomedicine*, in contrast to earlier forms of medical knowledge and discourse. Second, and closely related, it would be equally easy to assume that the identification of the condition's genetic basis would result in an essentially reductionist approach to diagnosis, with a concomitant simplification in the description and categorization of the condition itself. New genetic technologies might, according to this account, remove ambiguities of clinical medicine and create a stable set of disease classifications and we have seen this in the field's response to the development of the MECP2 test.

Our understanding of Rett syndrome – which we are treating as a case study of wider processes – suggests otherwise. While it is undeniable that medical genetics has led to significant changes in diagnosis and nosography, it does not result in wholesale transformations in the forms of medical knowledge and their reproduction. The simplification of diagnostic categories and diagnostic processes is itself part of a more complex trajectory. Classificatory systems and definitions of diseases characteristically go through cycles of explanatory accounts that veer between simplifying models and explanations that introduce greater complexity. Simplifications are associated with essentially reductionist accounts, in which clinical entities are attributed primarily or exclusively to single causes or systems (the immune system, viral infections, genetic causes and predispositions). There are, however, processes that tend towards greater complexity once more. In many cases, including Rett syndrome, the picture is not susceptible to simple, reductionist explanations. There are cyclical patterns of simplicity and complexity. They do not necessarily affect single disease entities at a time, but classes or families of conditions. The same explanatory framework, such as a genetic cause, can provide the basis for simplification *and* complexity, as scientific specializations – as well as their medical applications – can go through parallel processes of change. We have seen that the description of Rett syndrome as a genetic condition does not result in a purely reductionist account. In our examination of clinical consultations we have seen that clinical manifestations do not necessarily map unequivocally onto genetic findings, and vice versa.

Moreover, the nosology of disease classifications is not itself static. There are processes of reordering and shifting boundaries. Medical classifications are subject to continuous boundary changes (cf. Bowker and Star, 2000). These processes include recurrent cycles of *lumping and splitting*. Processes of lumping and splitting seem to be indigenous to many specialized and scientific domains of knowledge and practice and they have been widely documented. The lumping and splitting of medical entities is a recurrent feature of systems of medical classification. Within any one particular field or domain, there are tendencies towards the proliferation of entities – more and more finely discriminated classifications are identified. This appears to be an almost inherent feature of classificatory systems – or more properly of humans' creation and use of such systems. Splitting can create more and more types and subtypes, species and subspecies. Lumping, on the other hand, exploits a different principle that is equally an inherent property in classificatory systems. In principle, examples, cases and species can always be allocated to broader, more embracing, classificatory types. Such a process of 'lumping' thus minimizes the difference between local varieties and stresses broader family resemblances. We have seen that Rett syndrome in its recent history reflects these two tendencies simultaneously. While the identification of the MECP2 gene partly helps to resolve the identification of the syndrome, complexity is also increased when it expands the clinical picture and introduces new classificatory possibilities (such as 'Rett-like' conditions, patients with classic Rett but without the genetic mutation, or mutations with mutations in MECP2 but without the classic constellation of presenting signs and symptoms). Equally, aligning the syndrome to a wider spectrum of neurodevelopmental disorders affecting children and young people under the label autism spectrum disorders and pervasive developmental disorders (the American Psychiatric Association definition includes autism, atypical autism, Asperger and Rett syndrome) represents a possible 'lumping' and complicating direction in its developing trajectory.

It is, however, noticeable that the consequences of 'new' genetic medicine and the identification of genetic origins does not necessarily lead to wholesale changes in the classification and nosography of diseases and syndromes. Modern medicine and contemporary biomedical knowledge are heir to a classical nosology, based on a system of discrete, named entities. Many of these are longstanding in the inventory of clinical entities. Many were identified and named over the past 300 years or so. Others, of course, like Rett syndrome itself are of recent origin. Many of these named conditions have been subject to change – sometimes radical change – in terms of their explanations and treatments. Yet the array of named conditions themselves remains remarkably stable. Indeed, their status *as* entities remains given. Changing research or treatments may introduce quite major modifications in the description or management of the condition, yet the nomenclature and the nosology it supports remain resistant to change.

There is, therefore, in the trajectory of any given condition, an aspect of the trajectory we refer to as *saving the categories*. That is, a process of 'tinkering', of iterations of amendments and modifications, to bring successive measurements, models and causes into line with the prevailing classificatory scheme. This process can lead to elaborations on the underlying model, with a proliferation of variants and modifications. In the biomedical field, the underlying model(s) that must be safeguarded include the 'classic' descriptions of clinical entities (the categories). These can be modified and adjusted in order to accommodate changing diagnostic and investigative practice, new technologies, new therapeutic regimes and so on. This process does not automatically result in wholesale changes and paradigm shifts in the clinical categories, but in a series of small changes 'tinkering' with the existing categories. This process, with sometimes multiple iterations, provides for an especially characteristic feature of clinical medicine. That is, the capacity to express changing knowledge bases against a backdrop of apparently great stability in its underlying classificatory system. In other words, we do not repeatedly get 'new' conditions as underlying pathology is elucidated and modified. Rather, we witness elaborations and variants of existing classificatory systems.

Equally, our arguments about trajectories, stability and change are not subsumed under grand narratives of paradigm changes in medicine and the biomedical sciences more widely. There have been several such narratives that variously periodize the rise and development of modern and contemporary medicine. Such periodizations and narratives are normally intended to demonstrate that there is a recent and current epoch that is designated in terms of biomedicine, biomedicalization or some equivalent designation. First, we are not convinced by arguments that imply successive stages in medical or biomedical thought and we are certainly *not* persuaded of the suggestion of discrete epochs of medical and scientific practice, each supplanting the previous one. The trajectories of individual conditions are complex and variable.

Second, insofar as they are identifiable, different modes of medical perception and practice are not mutually exclusive. We do not observe, say, the 'molecular gaze' supplanting the 'clinical gaze', for instance. Biomedical knowledge does not replace classical clinical practice. The laboratory does not supplant the clinic. Insofar as we can discern different modes of understanding or practice, they do not add up to an unfolding evolutionary narrative. If anything they form multiple palimpsests. Different modes of medical understanding co-exist and may be in play simultaneously in the same clinical setting. In the same way, it is vital to note that while we describe 'trajectories' of medical conditions, the same general principle still holds. Successive 'versions' of diseases and syndromes may also be in play simultaneously. We may have to think of multiple versions unfolding over time, but in principle remaining 'in play' simultaneously. We are, therefore, likely to encounter multiple and competing versions of any given condition at any given time. Our own approach is rather different. While we acknowledge that new forms and sources of knowledge have brought in their train major changes in medicine – discoveries in genetics prominent among them in recent years – we believe that it is misleading to think of these in terms of successive waves or periods of change, each supplanting the previous one. We elaborate on these observations in the sections that follow.

The clinic's multiple births and deaths

Our book is one in a long tradition of ethnographic studies of the clinic, of medical knowledge and of distinctive modes of medical perception. A number of commentators have reflected on the parallels between the 'clinical gaze' and the 'ethnographic gaze'. For instance, Lawlor (2003: 31) suggests that:

> Gazing ... conveys the interrelatedness of theory and practice. In both clinical practice and ethnography, the eye is directed by an agenda that incorporates theoretical sensitivities toward where one might look, what one should see, what is foregrounded, where attention should go, and how long attention should linger. Gaze is theory driven, even when in a particular research mode the theory orienting the eye is one of attempting to free the mind from a particular theoretical stance or preconceived notions.

The clinic is always in transition. It is always poised between tradition and modernity. Through these transformations, the clinic always obeys its own distinctive mode of apperception and reasoning. The clinic therefore stands for two things simultaneously: it is out of time, and it is caught up in a frantic process of renewal and change. As well as the features of tradition and change, the clinic has another dual existence, it is simultaneously the concrete lived reality of medical knowledge and practice *and* an idea. 'The clinic' as an object of the imagination is just as important as the specific detail of actual medical work in any given institution, in any particular historical epoch. In discussing the idea of the clinic we are critical of a series of major authors who have not realized, perhaps, that the historical specificities and unique configurations that they claim to identify are in fact just another in a series of representations of the clinic. Historical–sociological discussions of the clinic can be read, therefore, as a kind of cyclical mythology, repeating the same formulae, finding the same innovations repeatedly.

We use the specific, concrete example of Rett syndrome, as well as our previous work on dysmorphology generally, to discuss the role of the clinic in contemporary medicine. We do so in order to address the broader intellectual agenda posed by successive commentaries on clinical medicine and the role of technological innovation. The recent trajectory of Rett syndrome has, as we have already described, become one of the many conditions for which a genetic basis has been identified. It thus provides a perfect case study for the broader trajectory whereby a condition becomes geneticized, and – more broadly still – a trajectory in which a clinically defined condition is provided with an innovative, technologically defined classification. We therefore develop our argument in relation to Rett syndrome in order to test the extent to which genetics and other technologies successively supplant the clinic, to examine the intersections of the clinic and the laboratory and to trace some of the consequences of that trajectory. We shall retrace some classic formulations of the clinic, its features and its multiple 'deaths'.

While by no means novel in this context, the work of Michel Foucault is an especially useful pivot, about which to gain some leverage on this topic. Foucault's account of the emergence of a distinctively modern clinic is to be founding his monograph *Naissance de la clinique*, first published in 1963 and published in English as *The Birth of the Clinic* a decade later (1973). Foucault's book is about the emergence of a distinctive mode of medical understanding, practice and perception in Paris in the post-Revolutionary period. Its strength lies in the deployment of a number of key insights into medical understanding; its weakness is to universalize a constellation of features that had different historical trajectories beyond Paris.

In Foucault's analysis, there is a radical rupture between the medicine of the eighteenth century in France and the revolutionary medicine of Paris. The eighteenth-century regime of medical knowledge is characterized as a medicine of symptoms – the patient's descriptions and experiences of ill-health. The physical signs of disease are not regarded as important. The eighteenth-century practice and theory of medicine Foucault represents as a nosography that is a kind of natural history.

This nosography is essentially a *classification* of diseases, often couched in highly generalized explanatory frameworks, which are in turn frequently grounded in general *systems* of classificatory principles. In this natural-historical version of medicine, diseases manifest themselves in the patient, but are not necessarily anchored in particular bodily organs or anatomical systems. The manifestation of a disease in a given individual patient is understood as the playing out of the natural progression of the disease. In the course of this development, the disease itself can migrate around the body. The work of the clinician resides primarily in fitting symptoms to the classificatory system, from which is derived a regimen of treatment. This is a medicine of symptoms more than signs.

The early nineteenth century, on the other hand, sees the emergence of several features that contribute to a revolutionary, radical disjuncture. This version of events is, of course, indebted to Foucault's more general methodology, in that it is based on a radical rupture between modes of knowledge. The key features that Foucault identifies for the revolutionary period are:

1. The first is the development of morbid anatomy, or clinical pathology. The post-mortem examination of the dead, diseased body is a crucial element in this modern system of medical knowledge. The symptoms of the patient's illness can now be correlated with specific pathological manifestations – lesions, tumours and other tissue damage – located and localized to particular organs.
2. New clinical technology encourage the exploration of the interior workings of the patient's body. The stethoscope and the clinical thermometer allow for the medicated inspection of the interior. Symptoms – the subjective experience of the patient – can now be translated into signs that are warranted by the observing physician.

3. The hospital takes on a new significance in the system of medicine and the production of medical knowledge. It is no longer a repository of sick indigent populations. It is increasingly a site for the practice of specialized medicine. The hospital consultant becomes an elite practitioner.
4. The instruction of medical students on the wards of the hospitals means that medical knowledge and its reproduction is achieved in the highly localized space of the individual patient's bedside, as well as the dissecting room and the pathology section. The teaching hospital is thus constituted as a kind of living museum of pathology.

It is this institutional and technological context that gives rise to a distinctive mode of medical knowledge. Or, more precisely, it makes possible a new form of warrant for medical knowledge. This is what Foucault calls the 'clinical gaze' (although the English phrase is not an ideal one). The clinical gaze is founded on the assumption of a privileged perception. The clinician at the bedside becomes the repository of special powers of observation and inference. Just as the disease becomes localized in the body's organs, so the recognition of disease gets localized in the personal qualities of the clinician.

This attitude – the privileged status of the clinical gaze – is enhanced by various ceremonials of the teaching hospital that actually pre-date the revolutionary period. The teaching round is conducted by a senor clinician, in which the huddle of students is led round the wards in order to inspect patients and their conditions. The old tradition of the round is given renewed vigour and significance when the authority of clinical surveillance is enhanced.

The birth of the clinic thus grounds a new form of medical knowledge in the spectacular display of clinical material, arranged in the teaching hospital, exposed to the gaze of the clinician and the medical student, who visit and inspect the patient. The bedside is a site of privileged knowledge. Foucault's was by no means the first historical contribution to identify the emergence and significance of the modern clinic as a site of a new spatial and epistemological mapping of the patient's body, its constituent organs, and pathological processes (cf. Philo, 2000). Foucault was influenced directly by the work of Georges Canguilhem (1978). Canguilhem's monograph is primarily an exercise in medical epistemology, and is a kind of debate with the ghost of Bernard. Bernard's spirit of positive, experimental science leads him to assert that the pathological is to be understood in terms of an extrapolation of measured values from the normal state to abnormal states. The pathological is always to be understood in terms of excess or deficiency, as defined by the range of normal values, observed in the normally functioning body, and defined by positive, experimental science. Canguilhem uses Bernard and other French physiologists as a case study to argue something more general. He asserts, contrary to the French physiologists, that the pathological is not reducible to extrapolation from the normal. He argues that the pathological is qualitatively rather than mainly quantitatively different from normal physiology. Hence, Canguilhem argues that the clinic is not reducible to physiology, or to other sciences of normal biology. Pathological states, or disease entities, are, Canguilhem argued, *sui generis*: a different class of phenomena from those produced by the basic clinical sciences.

The French sociologists Jamous and Peloille (1970) take as their origin precisely the same teaching hospitals and modes of perception. The leaders of medicine in early nineteenth-century Paris were the social elite, highly selected through the university system and competitive examinations. They occupied the intellectual high ground. They had access to elite medical knowledge and perception as clinicians, exercising the clinical gaze, obsessed with post-mortem examinations. For about 50 years in the French university hospitals, knowledge and academic status coincided. But – and this is the key point in *their* account – Jamous and Peloille argue that this congruence of elite clinical status and the unquestioned supremacy of clinical knowledge was under assault: from physiology (Claude Bernard) and from bacteriology (Louis Pasteur).

In the later nineteenth-century French medical system, therefore, Jamous and Peloille identify a tension between different segments of the occupation. This is simultaneously a tension between status groups and between different knowledge systems. Clinicians felt their expertise and their standing assailed. They reaffirmed both simultaneously by affirming or reasserting the centrality of clinical knowledge based on a distinctive mode of understanding. They thus stressed varieties of *tacit* clinical knowledge, related to personal qualities such as experience, talent, intuition and gifts. Knowledge is thus warranted as personal and biographically grounded in the personal authority of the clinician. Hence, 'the clinic' becomes not merely the site of clinical work, but further affirmed as the origin of a distinctive mode of knowledge, and is contrasted with the impersonal warrant of laboratory-based experimental science.

Now this is a very durable and persistent mode of medical knowledge-warrant. In his classic contribution to the sociology of medicine, Freidson identified what he called the 'clinical mentality' (Freidson, 1970). The clinical mentality informs a medical practitioner who is pragmatic, relies on her or his *own* first-hand experience, stresses the significance of tacit knowledge, and believes that such knowledge has an indeterminate quality, irreducible to formula or explicit precept. It is marked by a degree of scepticism concerning scientific evidence, or scientific theory – always evaluating it against the touchstone of experience. The clinical mentality is, therefore, intensely personal as well as scientific, biographical as well as institutional. This does not mean that clinicians pay no heed to evidence derived from journal science, or from laboratory work. That, of course, would be absurd. But it does mean that 'the clinic' is inhabited and informed by multiple discourses and sources of authority. The personal authority of the clinician synthesizes them, draws on them pragmatically and differentially, evaluates them against personal knowledge, and always does so against the background of experience.

Now this repeated, or possibly cyclical, pattern of practices and knowledge-claims has continued. There have been repeated examples of how claims are made that new scientific methods and findings radically transform not just the content of the medical knowledge, but also its fundamental character. The emergence of new science is repeatedly held to diminish the significance of the clinic and to transform the fundamental character of medical perception, decision-making and the value of disease entities themselves. Equally, such incursions from the laboratory are represented as constituting threats to the autonomy of the clinician. The epistemological assault on the clinic, according to some models, does not reside solely in the laboratory sciences. It is also driven by other forms of decontextualized knowledge, such as systems of regulation, treatment guidelines and protocols.

Before considering these recent and current perspectives, we want to return to Foucault's model for a moment. He locates the emergence of modern clinical medicine at the very end of the eighteenth and beginning of the nineteenth centuries. Now it comes as no great surprise that his is a thoroughly Paris-centred account. But if we look elsewhere, we find eighteenth-century medical practice and education that is more recognizably 'modern' than the image a natural-history nosography would seem to imply. If we look at Leiden rather than Paris, for instance, we see the 'modern' clinic of the physician and teacher Boerhaave. Indeed, Boerhaave's protégés took Leiden clinical knowledge and medical education to many centres of excellence. There was regular traffic between Leiden and Edinburgh, for instance, while physicians trained in that school also went to the USA. It is, in terms of historical accuracy, wrong to place too much faith in Foucault's account. As with most of his work, his own insistence on discontinuities leads him to exaggerate the revolutionary changes and the differences between one medical epoch and another. It is wrong for Foucault's readers to assume that his highly confined 'genealogy' can be taken as a general history. The emergence of a modern clinic and its associated modes of perception, instruction and inference have a longer duration, are more gradual and patchy, and take place at different sites at different rates. Indeed, what we really ought to learn is that 'the clinic' is a longstanding and durable mode of organization. The 'clinical mentality' is an enduring one. Lester King's historical and philosophical essay on medical knowledge represents a parallel development to the Parisian (King, 1982). He emphasizes the continuity of clinical reasoning, as a recurrent and fundamental mode of medical work and thought.

The clinic, then, seems permanently poised between tradition and innovation, between the *longue durée* of its core characteristics and rapidly changing scientific knowledge. Recent statements concerning the wholesale transformations of biomedicine mark yet another series of claims concerning the clinic. Like others before them, such claims seem premature at best. When authors like Haraway (1991) pronounce the 'death of the clinic' they recapitulate earlier, equally oversimplified, accounts of the transformation of medical work and knowledge. There is no doubt that within particular medical specialties, and in relation to specific conditions, new scientific procedures and new technologies can have profound implications for understandings of causation, the classification of disease entities, the description of pathology and opportunities for treatment. It is not the case, however, that 'the clinic' is thereby made redundant or that the clinical mentality is obliterated.

There remains in recent and contemporary medicine an essential tension between the perceptual and influential logic of the clinic and the work of the laboratory. Indeed, the clinical culture has, since whatever origins we ascribe, assimilated knowledge from 'elsewhere' with knowledge grounded in the here-and-now of the patient's body at the bedside. The presenting symptoms and the patient's subjective experience – the symptoms – have always been synthesized with pathological findings and physiological measurements. In Foucault's Paris the primary source of such 'scientific' evidence was the post-mortem examination that permits the correlation of bedside observation with specific pathology and the localization of disease in identifiable organs. Subsequent generations of medical practitioners have progressively synthesized the products of clinical pathology, histology, haematology and other disciplines of classifying and counting, together with the visualization techniques of X-rays, computed tomography scans, magnetic resonance imaging scans and the like (see, for instance, Saunders, 2008).

It would be equally absurd to imply that clinical medicine remains unaffected by changes in biological and medical sciences. There are plenty of examples in the published sociology, anthropology and history of medical knowledge to illustrate how diagnostic categories and aetiological theories are overturned by particular scientific changes. This perspective is exemplified by Christine Sinding's (1991) history of rickets. Sinding traces how the clinical entity 'rickets' has been transformed at various key junctures. In the nineteenth century, it presented as a bone disease associated with the loss of strength and susceptibility to infection. By the end of the nineteenth century rickets seemed like a complete disease: an aetiology defined as nutritional deficit, a clinical picture of soft, deformed bones; empirical treatment was with cod liver oil. But after 1920 nutritionists questioned the apparently simple cause of rickets. Vitamin D deficiency was not sufficient to capture the aetiology. Deficiency in phosphorous or calcium – or even a disturbance in the interaction between the two – could produce rickets-like symptoms in laboratory animals. The developing science of vitamin D itself made the nosological entity 'rickets' more complex again, not least when vitamin D-resistant rickets was identified. In other words, the very nature of rickets – notwithstanding the fact that it was well described and apparently well understood – has been transformed. Moreover, as Sinding makes clear, the contributions of laboratory science do *not* necessarily render the aetiology or nosology of a disease more simple or more clear. As in the case of rickets, the science complicated the clinical identification of the disease and its treatment.

There is, therefore, no need to assume, still less to conclude, that the laboratory sciences progressively replace clinical, experiential or tacit knowledge with reductionist explanations. On the contrary, there can be an interaction between clinical perception and judgment on the one hand, and the research findings of the laboratory. The laboratory rarely provides a 'gold standard' that substitutes for the clinic. Rather, we are likely to find that there is a process of formulation and reformulation of clinical entities that draws differentially and at different times on clinical and extra-clinical forms of knowledge. This is a theme illustrated by

Wailoo's (1997) account of the development of haematology in the twentieth century. The case of pernicious anaemia illustrates his general point. As a clinical entity, the identity of pernicious anaemia has varied over time, reflecting changing treatment regimes, the involvement of different medical specialties, as well as commercial interests. The condition has been identified in terms of the investigative and treatment technologies available for it. Successive medical technologies are active in constituting the clinical entity. They do not merely reveal a stable entity, therefore, but help to create the conditions for its existence as a distinct category.

So in reflecting on the models of the clinic and its tensions, we have to remember that it is not simply a matter of the clinic *or* the laboratory, or even of the clinic *and* the laboratory. The clinic and its modes of knowledge are always enmeshed in wider organizational contexts, divisions of labour, monetary interests and the like. New science and new technologies do not simply 'appear' and do not innocently transform or impinge on clinical knowledge. New medical technologies derive from commercial and industrial interests. Knowledge is mediated by mechanisms that are corporate products. The international distribution of new technologies – including treatments such as drugs – creates conditions of standardization and the calibration of techniques, reassessments and definitions that can transcend the dispersed, local arrangement of clinicians and their 'firms'. If we remain briefly with the topic of haematology, for example, then we can see how the development of the automated blood cell counter could lead to a widespread codification of practices in reviewing blood smear data, categorizing cases or establishing normal values (cf. Atkinson, 1995). Technologies readily become quasi-agents in shaping work practices and forming/framing medical classifications. But equally, clinicians are active in interpreting and using technologies. It is clear that the clinic is not susceptible merely to reductionist, technologically determined practices.

Despite strong pressures from bureaucratic and political interests to impose various gold standards, protocols, clinical guidelines and similar kinds of prescriptive machinery, they never succeed in determining clinical practice. This recurrent observation is documented amply by Timmermans and Berg (2003). Their research monograph brings together the results of several studies of evidence-based medicine and standardization in contemporary regimes of health care in the Netherlands and the USA. In the case study most directly relevant to our interests, a series of depth interviews with hospital doctors in paediatrics, they demonstrate how evidence-based medicine is refracted through the practical, clinical interests-at-hand of the doctors, and by their professional experience. The residents (hospital doctors) affirmed that the experience and personal authority of their medical superiors outweighed any research-based evidence that the more junior physicians might be able to assemble and bring to bear: 'Wherever we turn, the formal tools of EBM [evidence-based medicine] seem to run into a barrier of clinical judgement and experience. Research-based knowledge seems to perpetually fall short in clinical decision making. Residents refer to the extra quality needed as "experience", "competence" or "confidence"' (Timmermans and Berg, 2003: 163).

Timmermans and Berg are at pains to point out that the introduction of clinical guidelines, protocols and the like does *not* produce a linear evolutionary process in which medical practice is progressively rationalized and rendered increasingly 'scientific'. Equally, they do not wish to suggest simply that medical practice remains completely untouched by standardization, guidelines, protocols and evidence-based practice. Rather, they point out that there is a dynamic, shifting relationship between *definitions* of medical practice, as generated by scientific, bureaucratic, corporate and other frameworks, and the mundane, practical work of clinical decision-making, treatment and disposal. In the study of paediatric residents, for instance, Timmermans and Berg pointed out that resident physicians do not reject or ignore evidence-based medicine, but actively adapt and interpret the research evidence:

> A physician starts with a recommendation and adds qualifications to consider whether the guideline applies to this particular patient, ward, attending, time frame and resources. The generation of clinical judgement allows residents to apply protocols to patients for whom it was not intended because they gained insights with the rationale behind the evidence. It also facilitates skipping or substituting steps, working around the protocols, and appropriating them. The resident interacts with the protocols and guidelines' (Timmermans and Berg, 2003: 164).

The intense socialization of physicians, through the oral traditions and ceremonials of the clinic, again enforces the value of personal authority, localized knowledge and practical action.

This is the picture created in Atkinson's (1995) ethnography of knowledge-creation and reproduction among haematologists in the UK and the USA. This demonstrates how the practical work of defining disease entities, allocating cases to nosographic categories and deciding on treatment regimens are all managed through a number of interpretive frames and rhetorics of justification. What Elliot Mishler (1984) called 'the voice of medicine' is inhabited by several contrasting 'voices' – sometimes in competition, sometimes complementary. The voice of personal authority and experience alternates with the voice of journal science. Personal knowledge and professional status coincide in the synthesis of *clinical experience*.

Looked at from these perspectives, then, we can again see the persistence of the clinic as a distinctive site of knowledge production. New technologies, new scientific evidence, new regimes of guidance and accountability – these all transform the contexts of clinical work and the rhetorics of evaluation of clinical accountability. They do not, however, substitute for the clinic. The clinic, then, resists reductionism. New science can transform or reconfigure the disease entities with which the clinic deals; it can introduce new sources of evidence. Importantly, it can help transform the classifications of nosography: new entities are produced; old entities are fragmented; entities are reclassified; some diseases cease to exist for all practical, medical purposes. But these processes are, clinically speaking, always under-determined. The clinic is never, as it were, erased under the guise of scientific reductionism.

Now this is the general argument that we bring to bear on the nature of genetic medicine. The extraordinary development of genetic medicine in recent years is an important case in point: the intersection of the clinic, and the clinician's gaze, with changes in medical and biomedical science at the molecular level. It is easy to assume that genetic science might so transform the diagnosis and classification of disease as to render the clinic all but redundant. Indeed, some commentators have gone so far as to announce, or to predict, the death of the clinic, and its epistemological collapse into biomedical science. However, as we have seen in the Rett clinic, the realities of genetic medicine and the consequences of new genetic science (in this case the MECP2 genetic test) for medical practice remain much more complex, and remain grounded in the forms of the clinic, its visual imagination, and the liturgies of its performance.

The biomedicalization thesis

The most recent contribution to debates concerning the periodization of medical knowledge and practice is the 'biomedicalization' thesis. In essence, this argues that the most recent period of medical history has witnessed a major transformation, and that we are currently witnessing *biomedicalization*. Clarke *et al.* (2003) provide one clear example of this position. Their discussion is based on perceived changes in the organization and knowledge-base of American medicine. The authors argue that the twenty-first century is witnessing a paradigmatic change in medicine:

> Biomedicalization is our term for the increasingly complex, multi-sited, multidirectional processes of medicalization that today are being both extended and reconstituted through the emergent social forms and practices of a highly and increasingly technoscientific biomedicine (p. 162).

This general transformation is held to reflect changes in organizational structures, informational resources and technical resources.

The phase of biomedicalization, it is argued, supplants that of medicalization, which in turn replaces a period of classic medical knowledge and practice. Medicalization supplants the classical phase at about the time of the Second World War in this model, and biomedicalization emerges from about 1980 onwards. There are many constituent strands to this supposed transformation. For our purposes, the changes in the practice of clinical medicine are significant. The focus of the classical period is said to be on acute illnesses, and the main mode of clinical action is the exercise of clinical skill or surgical intervention. The period of 'medicalization', on the other hand, is characterized by chronic conditions, accompanied by the routinization of medical care and surveillance. Biomedicalization is founded on a concentration on risk and health, with a main mode of action enacted through drugs and techno-devices. The dominant mode of scientific knowledge in the classical period is that of germ theory, that of the post-war period of medicalization is dominated by ideas derived from biochemistry and pharmacology, while the period of biomedicalization reflects the rise of nanotechnologies and biotechnologies. The current, biomedicalized period is therefore characterized in terms of the molecularization and geneticization of medical knowledge, with a corresponding reliance on a digital infrastructure.

Now in these and similar general schemas, it is always hard to pin down specific and concrete examples of what might count as 'biomedicalization' as opposed to 'medicalization'. It is also hard to avoid the implication that this historical movement is driven by a form of technological determinism, for all that its authors disclaim such an analysis. It is, moreover, hard to avoid the implication in this historical narrative that one 'era' of medicine supplants and erases previous ones. It is, however, our contention that this would be a mistake – whether or not the authors of the biomedicalization thesis intend it.

In fact, what is interesting about the development of medical knowledge and diagnostic practice is *not* that it is characterized by successive modes of action, each suppressing the former. We should certainly not think of medicine as a series of discrete moments or epochs. Whatever the merits of a Foucauldian perspective, we should also be wary of exaggerated claims concerning ruptures and revolutions in medical thought. 'Earlier' modes of thought and practice are remarkably resilient. The modes of perception and reasoning associated with the classical period of medicine – indeed, some of those associated with pre-modern forms – persist. To be sure, they are supplemented by new modes of investigation, such as diagnostic or predictive genetic tests, new imaging techniques (cf. Saunders, 2008), and other forms of 'laboratory' investigation. This is, indeed, a long process. The history of medical inference is the history of successive innovations in investigative techniques, whether it be in the staining and inspection of cells, the development of haematological investigations, the rise of immunology, or other technological innovations.

But rather than thinking of successive epochs, or periods, we should think more in terms of a *palimpsest* of knowledge-forms, techniques and practices. A palimpsest is a text that has been overwritten on one or more occasions, so that more than one text can be read from it simultaneously. Contemporary medicine is best thought of as a palimpsest: multiple modes of knowledge-production and clinical practice are inscribed in it. Depending on circumstance and context, different modes of knowledge-in-use may be mobilized. The classical clinic retains its enduring forms and modes of production. It is supplemented and overlaid with repeated technological innovations. The 'clinical gaze' is augmented by the use of imaging. The machinery of diagnostic inference is informed by protocols and risk-assessments. The tacit knowledge on which clinicians draw is modified by evidence-based medicine. But 'the clinic' endures. As we have argued, it would, therefore, we quite wrong to assume that the advent of genetic medicine implies a purely biomedicalized version of medical work. There is, however, a tendency to equate the recent rise of genetic medicine and post-genomic science with a postmodern condition that implies a post-clinical mode of reasoning and action.

It is our contention in the course of this book that even where we are dealing with significant innovations in genetic medicine, the 'older' forms of the clinic, in its classic sense and in its 'modern' sense too, remain powerful means of medical work and interpretation. In pursuing this line of argument we provide a critique of and a counterbalance to overheated claims concerning the wholesale transformation of medical work. Whatever the appeal of models of global innovation and the worldwide distribution of digital information, we must not lose sight of the fact that they remain always dependent on the *local* production of medical knowledge. While information about a condition (such as Rett syndrome) may circulate between international research collaborations, and within national networks of expertise, that 'information' itself is assembled out of a multitude of local, personal judgments. However much practitioners may seek to generate agreed global standards for the description and diagnosis of medical conditions, they are inevitably derived from local interpretations, and are in turn subject to local interpretation. Consequently, whatever the force of biomedicalization, or recurrent changes in biomedical 'platforms', these newer forms inscribe the outcomes of clinical work and the work of the clinic. Successive innovations bear within them their origins in the clinic, which are never altogether transcended.

The transformations of patienthood

Claims concerning the births and deaths of the clinic are also linked to narratives concerning the medical construction of patienthood. Just as the narratives of technoscientific change imply a transformed – often reduced – medical practitioner, so too do they imply a transformation in patienthood.

The 'patient' in contemporary, biomedicalized medicine is portrayed primarily in terms of a constellation of factors that help construct new kinds of biomedical identities. They include an emphasis on 'risk' rather than overt disease, the imperative for people to act as responsible consumers of health care, and as morally responsible for their own care (cf. Clarke *et al.*, 2003). These transformations in turn imply not only individual responsibility, but also newly emergent phenomena such as 'biological citizenship' (e.g. Rose, 2006). From this perspective, the gaze of medicine is no longer directed at the *patient* but on the population, and of the non-symptomatic individual, through an imperative of self-surveillance on the part of responsible individuals, through the identification of risk factors and values, and through the promotion of health-promoting regimes. Biological citizenship thus rests on new forms of governmentality, it is claimed, that include transformations in personal identity, under the widened gaze of organized medicine.

The transformations of medicine that give rise to its molecularization and geneticization are central to this process of reconfiguration. The rise of genetic medicine in particular is held to produce key transformations in patienthood, and indeed in personhood. We have already made reference to the 'geneticization' thesis in general terms. We need to examine it in more detail here, as it relates specifically to the creation of personhood. It would be all too easy to assume that the progressive identification of more and more conditions with a genetic basis leads inexorably to the redefinition of persons in molecular terms, or the transformation of social relations into genetically defined categories of biological relatedness and shared risk.

Clearly there are indeed tendencies in that direction. The insertion of genetics into a broad array of medical conditions undoubtedly introduces new forms of self-awareness, and the identification of genetic risk has significant implications for individuals who are affected, or potentially affected, and members of their kin. Equally, however, we must be careful not to assume wholesale transformations in this domain. If there is a persistent *longue durée* for the clinic, then there are equally enduring forms of personhood and social relatedness. If medical practice is best thought of as a palimpsest of knowledge-systems and practices, then so too is personhood and so too are social relations.

The idea of biological/biomedical citizenship is a case in point. Promoted by authors such as Rose (2006; Novas and Rose 2000), this notion has a double valency. On the one hand, it implies that individual and collective identities are increasingly shaped by shared biomedical characteristics. They include shared genetic risk, characteristics defined by ethnicity, shared environmental exposure and an array of features that are simultaneously social and natural. In that sense the contemporary person is rendered increasingly *biological*. Gender, race, lifespan and other life-chances are increasingly identified in terms of biologically given predispositions. So too are character traits, moral character, mental health, even sociability itself. At the same time, however, such biological-cum-medical categories, such as those prescribed by genetic constitution, create the possibility for the emergence of new social formations and new bases for collective action. Biological citizenship may, therefore, imply *mobilization* in terms of shared interests that are defined in biomedical terms.

There are clearly issues and problems, some of them biologically defined, about which can coalesce alliances and networks, and from within which may emerge forms of activism and citizenship. They have been documented in key research publications (e.g. Epstein, 1998; Brown, 1997). Likewise, the emergence of new biomedical technologies can give rise to the appearance of new bases of regulation and surveillance. Programmes of screening (including commercial, private-sector firms offering screening) and predictive genetic testing, DNA databases, biobanks and other techniques can create the conditions for new types of regulatory regime. Indeed, the wider context of biotechnology and genetic science create multiple possibilities of forensic investigation, population screening, risk assessment, actuarial calculation, and the identification of individuals. These technologies can, in turn, be linked directly to matters of insurance, employability, entitlement to health care and other benefits, and security-based policing.

It would, however, be unwise to *assume* that because these possibilities exist, and because they are being realized in some contexts, there are wholesale transformations in identity-formation, or in regimes of governmentality, based on biomedical technologies and categories. Indeed, as several key sociological and anthropological studies have shown, involvement with genetic conditions does not lead inexorably to a geneticized identity, or to a 'master-status' defined primarily in biomedical terms.

One cannot assume, therefore, that the identification of an inherited condition in a family, or the identification of an inherited risk, or indeed the identification of carrier or mutation status, will automatically give rise to a transformation in personhood or patienthood. Moreover, one cannot assume that biomedical processes, such as diagnostic or predictive genetic testing, will entail wholesale transformations in the relationship of the 'patient' and the 'clinic'. The biomedicalization thesis holds that patienthood is changed, and that the classic sick role is superseded, in a movement from patienthood to the social position of the consumer of health care, responsible for health maintenance and subject to an extended form of medical surveillance. Our own research and that of others on a series of genetic conditions, suggests once again that this is not an inexorable process. A great many of the individuals and patients within this and our previous studies displayed a 'classic' orientation towards the clinic and towards the embodied authority of the medical practitioner.

Again, our own work with individuals and their family members leads us to suggest that everyday social life is not necessarily transformed by biomedicalizing processes. Family life is, of course, impacted on by the presence of clinical conditions. Severe developmental delay and problematic development caused by the wide array of genetic conditions known collectively as the clinical specialism 'dysmorphology', for instance, clearly create issues in everyday living, and give rise to a range of social and cultural issues for the parents of affected children. Likewise, haemophilia creates serious problems of everyday functioning, as well as creating issues of family members' genetic status (cf. Gregory *et al.* 2007). But members of families where there are affected individuals, or members who are themselves carriers or at risk are not thereby automatically 'geneticized' into novel forms of identity and biologically defined personhood. One cannot read off from highly generalized discourse-based accounts to everyday lives. The implications of biomedical innovation for patients, families and others are an empirical question. They are subject to local variation, cultural framing and interpersonal negotiation.

Equally, therefore, one must recognize that the construction and interpretation of clinical entities is not confined to the clinic or the laboratory. Families and domestic settings are themselves sites where everyday phenomena of heath and ill-health, diseases and syndromes, risks and prognoses are generated, shared (or not), interpreted (or not). It is for that reason that we treat 'the family' as a further site for the construction of the syndrome. While biological citizenship as a concept may overstate the case, we recognize that the persistence of the clinic – one of our key themes – implies the persistence of 'the patient'. That is, the persistence of a mode of thought that seeks to interpret the phenomena of medical conditions, within an interpretative framework of mundane reasoning, and that intersects with the clinical perceptions of the clinician in multiple ways.

In describing families as sites for the construction of a condition like Rett syndrome, we are *not* assuming from the outset that this necessarily constitutes what has sometimes been called 'lay expertise'. This latter phrase has given rise to a good deal of unhelpful controversy. There is no doubt that patients, carers and other individuals may cultivate a good deal of knowledge about a given condition. They experience or observe its trajectory; they can become sensitive to changes in symptoms and the presentation of the condition; they can achieve a close acquaintance with the body; they can grasp the impact of a medical condition on everyday living. They can also acquire knowledge and information about 'their' condition from public sources: the Internet provides a rich source of data for many people, including multiple sites explicitly designed for patients and their family members or carers. They can also – like anybody else – glean information from 'textbook' sources, including information aimed primarily at medical practitioners. In these and various other ways, therefore, they can become what Schutz called 'well-informed citizens', with a variety of types of knowledge and understanding. We make no prior assumptions concerning the status of that knowledge, nor do we adjudicate *a priori* whether it constitutes 'lay expertise'.

Equally, however, we recognize that patients and family members are by no means the passive victims of biomedicalization or geneticization. They are actively engaged in the interpretation of their condition. This does not mean, however, that we should automatically assume that they are therefore to be regarded as well-informed 'consumers' of their health care, or that they embrace a biological citizenship as active representatives of a neo-liberal market ideology.

The structure and functions of family knowledge are empirical issues. We do not end this account, therefore, with a general thesis concerning the status of such knowledge, and we make no equivalent assumptions concerning the actions of family members as interpreters of medical phenomena. We do, however, treat such knowledge seriously, in that it merits close analytic attention. This and our own previous research on the social contexts of genetic conditions, however, leads us to set aside any presuppositions based on genetic exceptionalism. The fact that a condition is identified as having a genetic origin does not necessarily mean a wholesale transformation in people's understandings of biological and social relatedness, on the understanding of inheritance and relations between the generations. We do not assume that genetic knowledge, or recent innovations in biomedical knowledge more generally, necessarily mean major changes in conceptualizations of the body, health, illness, disability and related phenomena.

References

Aase JM (1990) *Diagnostic dysmorphology*. New York, NY: Plenum Medical.

Amir RE, Van den Veyver IB, *et al.* (1999) Rett syndrome is caused by mutations in X-linked MECP2, encoding methyl-CpG-binding protein 2. *Nat Genet*, 23: 185–88.

Amir RE, Van den Veyver IB, Schultz R, *et al.* (2000) Influence of mutation type and X chromosome inactivation on Rett syndrome phenotypes. *Ann Neurol*; 47: 670–79.

Angelman H (1965) 'Puppet' children: A report of three cases. *Dev Med Child Neurol*, 7: 681–88.

Atkinson P (1995) *Medical talk and medical work: the liturgy of the clinic*. London: Sage.

Bazerman C (1981) What written knowledge does: Three examples of academic discourse. *Phil Soc Sci*, 11: 361–87.

Bharadwaj A (2002) Uncertain risk: genetic screening for susceptibility to haemochromatosis *Health, Risk & Society*, 4: 227–40.

Bharadwaj A, Atkinson P, Clarke A and Worwood M (2007) Medical classification and the experience of genetic haemochromatosis, in Atkinson P, Glasner P, and Greenslade H (eds) *New genetics, new identities*. London: Routledge.

Bluebond-Langner M (1980) *The private worlds of dying children*. Princeton, NJ: Princeton University Press.

Bowker GC and Star SL (2000) *Sorting things out: Classification and its consequences*. Boston, MA: MIT Press.

Brown MP (1997) *Replacing citizenship: AIDS activism and radical democracy*. New York, NY: Guildford Press.

Brown P (1995) Naming and framing: The social construction of diagnosis and illness. *J Health Soc Behavior*, 35: 34–52. Special issue: forty years of medical sociology: the state of the art and directions for the future.

Budden S (1986) Rett syndrome: studies of 13 affected girls. *Am J Med Genet*, 24: 99–109.

Canguilhem G (1978) *On the normal and the pathological*. Cohen RS (ed.), Fawcett CR (trans.). Dordrecht: Reidel.

Cartwright L (1995) *Screening the body: Tracing medicine's visual culture*. Minneapolis, MN: University of Minnesota Press.

Chen RZ, Akbarian S, Tudor M and Jaenisch M (2001) Deficiency of methyl-CpG binding protein-2 in CNS neurons results in a Rett-like phenotype in mice. *Nat Genet*, 27, 327–31.

Clarke A (1996) Rett syndrome. *J Med Genet*, 33: 693–99.

Clarke A, Shim J, Mamo L, *et al.* (2003) Biomedicalization: technoscientific transformations of health, illness, and U.S. biomedicine. *Am Sociolog Rev*, 68(2): 161–85.

Coleman M, Brubaker J, Hunter K and Smith G (1988) Rett syndrome: a survey of North American patients. *J Ment Defic Res*, 32: 117–24.

Colvin L, Leonard H, de Klerk H, *et al.* (2004) Refining the phenotype of common mutations in Rett syndrome. *J Med Genet*, 41: 25–30.

Davis AG and Strong PM (1976) Aren't children wonderful? A study of the allocation of identity in developmental assessment, in Stacey M (ed.), *The sociology of the National Health Service*. Monograph 22. Keele: University of Keele.

Davis JA, Naruse S, Chen H, *et al.* (1998) An Alzheimer's disease-linked PS1 variant rescues the developmental abnormalities of PS1-deficient embryos. *Neuron*, 20: 603–9.

Epstein S (1998) *Impure science: AIDS, activism, and the politics of knowledge*. Berkeley, CA: University of California Press.

Featherstone K, Latimer J, Atkinson P, *et al.* (2004) Dysmorphology and the spectacle of the clinic. *Sociol Health Illness*, 27: 551–74.

Featherstone K, Atkinson P, Bharadwaj A and Clarke AJ (2006) *Risky relations: family and kinship in the era of new genetics*. Oxford: Berg.

Fleck L (1979) *Genesis and development of a scientific fact*. Bradley F and Trenn TJ (eds), Trenn TJ and Merton RK (trans.). Chicago, IL: University of Chicago Press.

Foucault M (1973) *The birth of the clinic*. London: Tavistock.

Freidson E (1970) *Profession of medicine*. New York, NY: Dodd Mead.

Gill H, Cheadle JP, Maynard J, *et al.* (2003) Mutation analysis in the MECP2 gene and genetic counselling for Rett syndrome. *J Med Genet*, 40: 380–84.

Gregory M, Baddington P, Dimond R, Atkinson P, Clarke A, and Collins P (2007) Communicating about haemophilia within the family: the importance of context and of experience. *Haemophilia*, 2: 189–98.

Guy J, Hendrich B, Holmes M, *et al.* (2001) A mouse Mecp2-null mutation causes neurological symptoms that mimic Rett syndrome. *Nat Genet*, 27: 322–26.

Guy J, Gan J, Selfridge J, *et al.* (2007) Reversal of neurological defects in a mouse model of Rett syndrome. *Science*, 315: 1143.

Hagberg B (1991) Rett syndrome: clinical peculiarities, diagnostic approach, and possible cause. *Pediatr Neurol*, 5: 75–83.

Hagberg B, Aicardi J, Dias K and Ramos O (1983) A progressive syndrome of autism, dementia, ataxia, and loss of purposeful hand use in girls: Rett syndrome: report of 35 cases. *Ann Neurol*, 14: 471–79.

Hagberg B, Hanefeld F, Percy A and Skjeldal O (2002) An update on clinically applicable diagnostic criteria in Rett syndrome. Comments to Rett Syndrome Clinical Criteria Consensus Panel Satellite to European Paediatric Neurology Society Meeting. Baden Baden, Germany, 11 September 2001. *Eur J Paediatr Neurol*, 6: 293–97.

Haraway D (1991) *Simians, cyborgs, and women: the reinvention of nature*. London: Routledge.

Harper PS (1998) *Practical genetic counselling* 5th edn. Oxford: Butterworth-Heinemann.

Hoffbuhr K, Devaney JM, LaFleur B, *et al.* (2001) MeCP2 mutations in children with and without the phenotype of Rett syndrome. *Neurology*, 56: 1486–95.

Horton, A (2010) **IRSF** email newsletter, Feb.

Huppke P, Held M, Hanefeld F, *et al.* (2002) Influence of mutation type and location on phenotype in 123 patients with Rett syndrome. *Neuropediatrics*, 33: 63–68.

Jamous H and Peloille B (1970) Professions or self-perpetuating systems? Changes in the French university-hospital system, in Jackson JA (ed.), *Professions and professionalization*. Cambridge: Cambridge University Press.

Jones KL (1997) *Smith's recognizable patterns of human malformation*, 5th edn. Philadelphia, PA: WB Saunders.

Kammoun F, de Roux N, Boespflug-Tanguy O, *et al.* (2004) Screening of MECP2 coding sequence in patients with phenotypes of decreasing likelihood for Rett syndrome: a cohort of 171 cases. *J Med Genet*, 41: e85.

Kerr A and Stephenson JBP (1986) A study of the natural history of Rett syndrome in 23 girls. *Am J Med Genet*, 24(suppl 1): 77–83.

Kevles B (1997) *Naked to the bone*. New Brunswick, NJ: Rutgers University Press.

King L (1982) *Medical thinking: a historical preface*. Princeton, NJ: Princeton University Press.

Laccone F, Huppke P, Hanefeld F and Meins M (2001) Mutation spectrum in patients with Rett syndrome in the German population: Evidence of hot spot regions. *Human Mut*, 17: 183–90.

Latimer J, Featherstone K, Atkinson P, *et al.* (2006) Rebirthing the clinic: the interaction of clinical judgement and molecular technology in the production of genetic science. *Science, Technol Human Values*, 31: 599–630.

Lawlor MC (2003) Gazing anew: the shift from a clinical gaze to an ethnographic lens. *Am J Occupat Ther*, 57(1): 29–39.

London Dysmorphology Database (2000) version 2.2, Electronic Publishing. Oxford: Oxford University Press.

Mishler EG (1984) *The discourse of medicine: dialectics of medical interviews*. Norwood, NJ: Ablex.

Myers G (1990) *Writing biology: texts in the construction of scientific knowledge*. Madison, WI: University of Wisconsin Press.

Naidu S, Murphy M, Moser H and Rett A (1986) Rett syndrome – natural history in 70 cases. *Am J Med Genet*, 24(suppl 1): 61–72.

Novas C, Rose N (2000) Genetic risk and the birth of the somatic individual. *Econ Soc*, 29: 485–513.

Pelka GJ, Watson CM, Radziewic T, *et al.* (2006) Mecp2 deficiency is associated with learning and cognitive deficits and altered gene activity in the hippocampal region of mice. *Brain* 129: 887–98.

Philo C (2000) The birth of the clinic: an unknown work of medical geography. *Area*, 32(1): 11–19.

Pictures of Standard Syndromes and Undiagnosed Malformations (1991) (version 5.1). Melbourne: The Murdoch Institute for Research into Birth Defects.

Ramocki MB, Tavyev YJ and Peters SU (2010) The MECP2 duplication syndrome. *Am J Med Genet A*, 152A: 1079–88.

Rett A (1966) Uber ein cerebralatrophisches Syndrom bei Hyperammonamie. Vienna: Bruder Hollinek.

Rett A (1966) Uber ein eigenartiges hirnatrophisches Syndrom in Kindesalter. *Wien Med Wochenschr*, 116: 723–38.

Rett A (1977) Cerebral atrophy associated with hyperammonaemia, in Vinken PJ, Bruyn GW, in association with Klawans HL (eds) Metabolic and deficiency diseases of the nervous system II. Chapter 16. *Handbook of clinical neurology*, Vol. 26. Amsterdam: Elsevier/North Holland Biomedical Press.

Rett Syndrome Diagnostic Criteria Working Group (1988) Diagnostic criteria for Rett syndrome. *Ann Neurol*, 23: 425–28.

Rose N (2006) *The politics of life itself: biomedicine, power, and subjectivity in the twenty-first century*. Princeton, NJ: Princeton University Press.

Saunders BF (2008) *CT suite: the work of diagnosis in the age of noninvasive cutting*. Durham, NC: Duke University Press.

Schanen C, Houwink EJ, Dorrani N, *et al*. (2004) Phenotypic manifestations of MECP2 mutations in classical and atypical Rett syndrome. *Am J Med Genet*, 126A: 129–40.

Sforza T, Lenhoff H and Lenhoff S (2006) *The strangest song*. Amherst, NY: Prometheus Books.

Shahbazian M, Young JI, Yuva-Paylor LA, *et al*. (2002) Mice with truncated mecp2 recapitulate many Rett syndrome features and display hyperacetylation of histone H3. *Neuron*, 35: 243–54.

Shaw A, Latimer J, Atkinson P and Featherstone K (2003) Surveying slides: clinical perception and clinical judgement in the construction of a genetic diagnosis. *New Genet Soc*, 22(1): 3–19.

Sinding C (1991) *Le clinicien et le chercheur: des grande maladies de carence à la médicine moléculaire*. Paris: Presses Universitaires de France.

Timmermans S and Berg M (2003) *The gold standard: the challenge of evidence-based medicine and standardization in health care*. Philadelphia, PA: Temple University Press.

Timmermans S and Haas S (2008) Towards a sociology of disease. *Sociol Health Illness*, 30(5): 659–76.

Villard L (2007) MECP2 mutations in males. *J Med Genet*, 44: 417–23: 417.

Voysey M (1975) *A constant burden: the reconstitution of family life*. London: Routledge & Kegan Paul.

Wailoo K (1997) *Drawing blood: technology and disease identity in twentieth-century America*. Baltimore, MD: Johns Hopkins University Press.

Wanga Y, Liua W, Wadaa E, *et al*. (2005) Clinico-pathological rescue of a model mouse of Huntington's disease by siRNA. *Neuroscie Res*, 53(3): 241–49.

Weaving LS, Williamson SL, Bennetts B, *et al*. (2003) Effects of MECP2 mutation type, location and X-inactivation in modulating Rett syndrome phenotype. *Am J Med Genet*, 118A: 103–14.

Weaving LS, Ellaway CJ, Gecz J and Christodoulou J (2005) Rett syndrome: clinical review and genetic update. *J Med Genet*, 42: 1–7.

Webb T and Latif F (2001) Rett syndrome and the MECP2 gene. *J Med Genet*, 38: 217–23.

Woolf SH (2008) The meaning of translational research and why it matters. *JAMA*, 299(2): 211–13.

Index

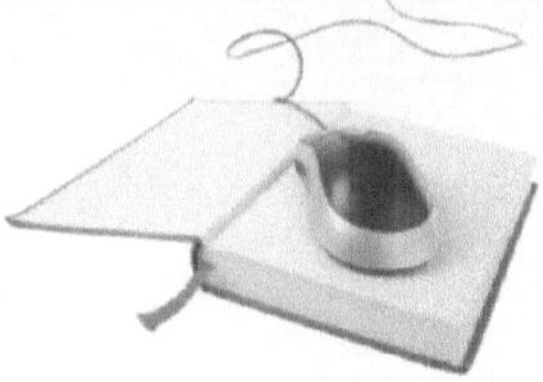